WORKBOOK TO ACCOMPANY

HUMAN DISEASES

Third Edition

D0164842

WORKBOOK TO ACCOMPANY

HUMAN DISEASES

Third Edition

Marianne Neighbors, EdD, RN
Professor
Eleanor Mann School of Nursing
University of Arkansas
Fayetteville, Arkansas

Ruth Tannehill-Jones, MS, RN
Chief Clinical Officer
Northwest Regency Hospital and Springdale Regency Hospital
Fayetteville & Springdale, Arkansas

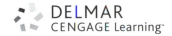
DELMAR
CENGAGE Learning

Australia • Brazil • Japan • Korea • Mexico • Singapore • Spain • United Kingdom • United States

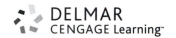
DELMAR
CENGAGE Learning

Workbook to Accompany Human Diseases, Third Edition
Marianne Neighbors and
Ruth Tannehill-Jones

Vice President, Career and Professional Editorial:
Dave Garza

Director of Learning Solutions:
Matthew Kane

Acquisitions Editor:
Matthew Seeley

Managing Editor:
Marah Bellegarde

Senior Product Manager:
Debra Myette-Flis

Editorial Assistant:
Samantha Zullo

Vice President, Career and Professional Marketing:
Jennifer McAvey

Executive Marketing Manager:
Wendy Mapstone

Senior Marketing Manager:
Kristin McNary

Marketing Coordinator:
Scott Chrysler

Production Director:
Carolyn S. Miller

Content Project Manager:
Thomas Heffernan

Senior Art Director:
Jack Pendleton

Library of Congress Control Number: 2009937494

ISBN-13: 978-1-4354-2753-2

ISBN-10: 1-4354-2753-X

Delmar
5 Maxwell Drive
Clifton Park, NY 12065-2919
USA

Cengage Learning is a leading provider of customized learning solutions with office locations around the globe, including Singapore, the United Kingdom, Australia, Mexico, Brazil, and Japan. Locate your local office at: **international.cengage.com/region**

Cengage Learning products are represented in Canada by Nelson Education, Ltd.

To learn more about Delmar, visit **www.cengage.com/delmar**

Purchase any of our products at your local college store or at our preferred online store **www.ichapters.com.**

Printed in the U.S.A.
4 5 6 7 12 11

CONTENTS

INTRODUCTION

Human Diseases, Third Edition, helps you learn basic disease information. Organized by body systems, this essential pathophysiology text is written specifically for allied health learners and as a reference for allied health professionals. This book is also ideal as a resource on basic diseases by anyone within the medical arena or lay community. It is designed to make difficult pathophysiology concepts easier to understand by using consistent organization, and it includes pronunciations, boxed features, and full-color illustrations and photos. Chapters progress through a basic review of anatomy and physiology before introducing the most common diseases. Common diseases and disorders are presented consistently through description, etiology, symptoms, diagnosis, treatment and prevention headings.

TO THE LEARNER

Each chapter in the workbook corresponds to the same chapter in the book. A variety of exercises are included to help reinforce the material you learned in the book. Types of exercises include matching; completion; short answer; true/false; defining terms, abbreviations, and diagnostic tests; and condition tables.

HUMAN DISEASES, THIRD EDITION, STUDYWARE™

Gain additional practice with the Study-Ware™ CD-ROM that offers an exciting way to enhance your learning of human diseases. The quizzes and activities are an interactive and engaging way to reinforce the content in the book. Review *How to Use Human Diseases, Third Edition, StudyWare™* in your book for a detailed description of this component.

WORKBOOK TO ACCOMPANY

HUMAN DISEASES

Third Edition

1

Concepts of Human Diseases

Introduction to Human Diseases

Define Terms

Define the following terms:

1. acute _____

2. auscultation _____

3. diagnosis _____

4. etiology _____

5. nosocomial _____

6. palliative _____

7. palpation _____

8. pathologic _____

9. symptom _____

10. mortality _____

Matching Terms

Match the following terms with the correct definition:

_____ 1. chronic   A. symptoms flare up or become worse

_____ 2. complication   B. a state of sameness

_____ 3. exacerbation   C. a disease that persists for a long time

_____ 4. homeostasis   D. the onset of a second disease or disorder

_____ 5. pathogens   E. removing a small piece of tissue for examination

                               F. microorganisms that cause disease

Match the following terms with the correct definition:

_____ 6. remission   A. predicted or expected outcome of the disease

_____ 7. pathologic   B. the study of tumors

_____ 8. disease   C. a change in structure or function

_____ 9. preventive   D. a time when symptoms are diminished

_____ 10. prognosis   E. something that reduces risk

                               F. caused by a disease

Define Abbreviations

Define the following abbreviations:

1. CBC _____

2. UA _____

3. CXR _____

4. EKG _____

5. CAT _____

Identify Diagnostic Tests

Define the following diagnostic tests:

1. Complete Blood Count _____

2. Urinalysis _____

3. Electrocardiography _____

4. Blood Glucose _____

5. Computerized Axial Tomography _____

Completion

Using the words in the list, complete the following statements:

acute	homeostasis
chronic	nosocomial
complication	palliative
diagnosis	predisposing factors
exacerbations	prognosis
holistic medicine	remission

1. _____ care is aimed at preventing pain and discomfort but does not seek to cure the disease.

2. The state of sameness or normalcy is known as _____.

3. A time when symptoms are diminished or temporarily resolved is called _____.

4. A condition that is short term with a sudden onset is called _____.

5. A problem arising from a prescribed treatment is called _____.

6. Risk factors are also called _____ _____.

7. _____ is the predicted or expected outcome.

8. Flare-ups or the return of symptoms is _____.

9. When the physician identifies or names a disease identified in a patient it is called the patient's _____.

10. Diabetes is a _____ disease because it lasts for a long or extended period of time.

11. A disease acquired from the hospital environment is called _____.

12. The concept where the whole person, rather than just the physical being, is considered is known as _____ medicine.

Short Answer

Provide answers to the following:

1. Define *predisposing* factors.

   _____

   _____

   _____

2. List some predisposing factors.

   a. _____

   b. _____

   c. _____

   d. _____

   e. _____

3. Explain the difference between a disorder and a syndrome.

   _____

   _____

   _____

   _____

4. Describe the pathogenesis of disease.

   _____

   _____

   _____

   _____

True / False

_____ 1. When using good handwashing techniques, you should use an antimicrobial soap.

_____ 2. It is important to use a fingernail cleaner whenever possible if you are following good handwashing protocol.

_____ 3. When washing the hands, after soaping and rubbing them, you should rinse starting from the wrist then over the fingertips.

_____ 4. The use of standard precautions is only recommended by the Centers for Disease Control and Prevention when administering care to a patient who is bleeding or has other body fluid discharge.

_____ 5. A hypodermic needle should never be recapped.

CASE STUDY

Emily is a 25-year-old Asian female. Emily is complaining of frequent headaches over the past 3 weeks. Emily is taking birth control pills and smokes one package of cigarettes a day. She complains of severe head pain, light sensitivity, nausea, and vomiting. She has had no relief from over-the-counter medications such as Tylenol or ibuprofen.

Using the information from the case study, list a possible diagnosis, risk factors, symptoms, and the etiology.

_____

_____

_____

_____

_____

_____

Mechanisms of Disease

Define Terms

Define the following terms:

1. congenital _____
_____

2. infection _____
_____

3. neoplasm _____
_____

4. malignant _____
_____

5. allergy _____
_____

6. cancer _____
_____

7. disease _____
_____

8. metastatic _____
_____

9. acute _____
_____

10. trauma _____
_____

Matching

Match the following terms with the correct definition:

_____ 1. hypertrophy   A. naming a disease

_____ 2. atrophy   B. increase in size or growth

_____ 3. diagnosis   C. without growth or decrease in cell size

_____ 4. gangrene   D. hypoxia of cells

_____ 5. ischemia   E. necrotic tissue attacked by saprophytic bacteria

                         F. enclosed in a capsule

Match the following terms with the correct definition:

_____ 6. infarct

A. a protective response triggered by injury

_____ 7. hypoxia

B. necrosis of cells due to ischemia

_____ 8. cachexia

C. proteins that react to antigens

_____ 9. antibodies

D. ill, thin, wasted appearance

_____ 10. inflammation

E. related to the small intestine

F. not enough oxygen in cells

Define Abbreviations

Define the following abbreviations:

1. TPN _____

2. AIDS _____

3. MVA _____

Completion

Using the words in the list, complete the following statements:

anorexia   infarct

benign   -itis

degenerative diseases   malignant

hypoxia   trauma

1. Diseases that are related to inflammation are identified by the suffix _____.

2. Neoplasms can be classified as _____ and _____.

3. Cellular injury and death may be due to _____, _____, or _____, or toxins or viruses.

4. When necrosis occurs due to ischemia, the area of dead cells is an _____.

5. Diseases related to aging may be called _____.

Short Answer

Provide answers to the following:

1. List the classification groups for trauma.

_____

_____

_____

2. State some examples of causes of diseases.

_____

_____

_____

3. Describe the following neoplasms:

adenoma _____

carcinoma _____

melanoma _____

sarcoma _____

4. Describe the changes in the body occurring in the aging process.

_____

_____

_____

5. What are the common ways the immune system may malfunction?

_____

_____

_____

6. List two ways the immune system protects the body.

_____

_____

_____

7. What factors affect the aging process?

a. _____

b. _____

c. _____

d. _____

e. _____

8. What conditions are necessary for a cell to survive?

a. _____

b. _____

c. _____

9. List the different types of cell adaptation.

a. _____

b. _____

c. _____

d. _____

e. _____

f. _____

10. What are the three different types of gangrene?

a. _____

b. _____

c. _____

True/False

_____   1. It is important to eat only small amounts of fiber in the daily diet.

_____   2. No more than one alcohol drink per day for females and two for male is the recommended daily allowance for a healthy lifestyle.

_____   3. Only moderate or small amounts of fat intake per day are recommended.

_____   4. The use of herbal remedies has been well known to be increasing among older persons.

_____   5. Consumers should be cautious in using herbal remedies, especially when combining them with other prescription medications.

CASE STUDY

Jonathan is a 29-year-old diesel mechanic. Because of the high cost of gasoline, Jonathan has been riding his motorcycle rather than his half-ton pickup back and forth to work in order to save money. The temperature is 95°F, so Jonathan decides not to wear his helmet on his way home from work. One mile down the freeway, Jonathan changes lanes and is hit by a car. He sustains a severe head injury. He is transported to the local hospital and admitted to the intensive care unit. Jonathan is unresponsive.

What criteria will be used to determine if Jonathan is brain dead?

_____

_____

_____

_____

_____

_____

_____

_____

_____

_____

_____

_____

CHAPTER 3

Neoplasms

Define Terms

Define the following terms:

1. benign _____

2. cachexia _____

3. cytology _____

4. hematoma _____

5. malignant _____

6. metastasis _____

7. neoplasm _____

8. palliative _____

9. preventive _____

10. tumor _____

Matching Terms

Match the following terms with the correct definition:

____ 1. biopsy	A. removing a small piece of tissue for microscopic examination
____ 2. carcinoma	B. something that corrects the disease or condition
____ 3. curative	C. determining the degree of differentiation of cells by microscopic examination
____ 4. dysplasia	D. neoplasm arising from epithelial tissue
____ 5. frozen section	E. technique that allows rapid diagnosis
	F. an alteration in size, shape, and organization of cells

Match the following terms with the correct definition:

____ 6. grading	A. an increase in cell number
____ 7. hyperplasia	B. the process of using light, short waves or x-rays
____ 8. radiation	C. neoplasm arising from connective tissue
____ 9. sarcoma	D. determining the degree of spread of a malignant tumor
____ 10. staging	E. a new growth
	F. determining the degree of differentiation of cells by microscopic examination

Identify Signs and Symptoms Of Cancer

Identify how the following may be signs or symptoms of cancer:

1. pain _____

2. obstruction _____

3. hemorrhage _____

4. anemia _____

5. fracture _____

6. infection _____

7. cachexia _____

Identify Diagnostic Tests

Match the following terms with the correct definition:

____ 1. screening
____ 2. occult stool
____ 3. annual physical examination
____ 4. cancer warning signals
____ 5. Pap test
____ 6. biopsy
____ 7. frozen section

A. microscopic exam that allows rapid diagnosis
B. measure, such as monthly breast and testicular exams
C. live tissue examination
D. yearly examination by physician
E. acronym CAUTION
F. staining test often used for cervical cytology
G. annual examination to screen for colon cancer

Completion

Using the words in the list, complete the following statements:

angiogenesis   cytology
biopsy   grading
carcinogens   hematoma
carcinoma in situ   staging
chemotherapy   tumors

1. _____ determines the degree of abnormality of the neoplasm.

2. A large tumor or swelling filled with blood, commonly called a bruise or contusion, is also known as a _____.

3. Neoplasms are commonly called _____.

4. Cancer-causing agents are known as _____.

5. _____ considers the degree of spread.

6. Removing a small piece of tissue for microscopic examination is known as a _____.

7. _____ is the examination of cells.

8. Atypical cells that just sit in the epithelial layer of tissue and have not broken through the basement membrane are called _____.

9. New growth of blood vessels is called _____.

10. _____ is the use of medications to kill or inhibit the growth of neoplasms.

Short Answer

Provide answers to the following:

1. Compare benign tumors to malignant tumors.

   _____

   _____

   _____

2. Explain the system used to classify neoplasms.

   _____

   _____

   _____

3. There are several factors that regulate the growth of normal cells. List them.

   a. _____

   b. _____

   c. _____

4. Describe a metastatic neoplasm.

   _____

   _____

   _____

5. What causes genetic mutation?

   a. _____

   b. _____

   c. _____

   d. _____

6. List the personal risk behaviors that put an individual at increased risk for developing cancer.

   a. _____

   b. _____

   c. _____

   d. _____

7. List the factors that decrease a female's risk for developing breast cancer.

   a. _____

   b. _____

   c. _____

8. Increased consumption of what dietary items is considered preventive in cancer development?

   a. _____

   b. _____

   c. _____

9. What are the American Cancer Society's recommendations for cancer prevention?

   a. _____

   b. _____

   c. _____

   d. _____

   e. _____

   f. _____

   g. _____

   h. _____

   i. _____

   j. _____

10. What does the acronym CAUTION stand for?

    C _____

    A _____

    U _____

    T _____

    I _____

    O _____

    N _____

11. What are the three major types of cancer treatment?

    a. _____

    b. _____

    c. _____

True / False

_____ 1. Beginning in their 20s, women should be made aware of the benefits and limitations of breast self-examinations (BSEs).

_____ 2. Finding a breast change means that cancer is present.

_____ 3. Researchers are testing the effectiveness of dendritic cell vaccines for preventing tumor growth and extending life in patients with cancer.

_____ 4. Dendritic cells occur naturally in tissues such as the skin and the lining of nose, lungs, stomach, and intestines.

_____ 5. Some studies have shown that alternative therapies used as the main treatment for breast cancer may result in increased recurrence of the disease and even death.

CASE STUDY

Susan is a 52-year-old elementary school teacher. Her sister (age 47) was recently diagnosed with metastatic breast cancer. Susan has yearly clinical breast exams and a mammogram but has never done a breast self-exam (BSE).

Describe the process of BSE as if you were explaining it to Susan.

_____

_____

_____

_____

CHAPTER 4

Inflammation and Infection

Define Terms

Define the following terms:

1. bacteria _____

    _____

2. trauma _____

    _____

3. hyperemia _____

    _____

4. adhesion _____

    _____

5. odoriferous _____

    _____

6. septicemia _____

    _____

7. pus _____

    _____

8. lesion _____

    _____

9. scab _____

    _____

10. purulent _____

    _____

Matching

Match the following terms with the correct definition:

_____ 1. pyogenic

_____ 2. abscess

_____ 3. cellulitis

_____ 4. fistula

_____ 5. keloid

A. a tract that connects two organs

B. movement of cells in response to chemicals

C. pus forming

D. excessive collagen formation

E. a localized collection of pus

F. inflammation of connective tissue

Match the following terms with the correct definition:

_____ 6. ulcer

_____ 7. infection

_____ 8. exudate

_____ 9. malaise

_____ 10. empyema

A. a crater-like lesion in the skin

B. a process of washing away necrotic tissue

C. fluid that seeps out of tissue or capillaries

D. invasion of microorganisms into tissue

E. an accumulation of pus in a body cavity

F. general ill feeling

Completion

Using the words in the list, complete the following statements:

abscesses

adhesions

cellulitis

dehiscence

inflammation

keloid

mast cells

primary union

skin testing

ulcers

1. _____ are also called tissue histocytes.

2. _____ is the nonspecific cellular and vascular reaction to tissue trauma.

3. Inflammatory lesions include _____, _____, and _____.

4. Healing by first intention is also called _____ _____.

5. Separation of tissue margins is called _____.

6. Excessive collagen formation often results in a hard, raised scar called a _____.

7. Fibrous bands that develop as a complication of surgery are called _____.

8. _____ may be used to determine the presence of exposure to a pathogen like TB.

Short Answer

Provide answers to the following:

1. Describe the basic defense mechanisms in the body that help prevent infections.

_____

_____

_____

2. Explain the steps in wound healing.

_____

_____

_____

3. List some common infectious microorganisms.

_____

_____

_____

4. What are the three primary goals of the inflammatory response?

    a. _____

    b. _____

    c. _____

5. What are the "foot soldiers" of the inflammatory process?

_____

_____

_____

6. Describe a lesion.

    a. _____

    b. _____

7. List three inflammatory lesions.

    a. _____

    b. _____

    c. _____

8. How is an abscess formed?

_____

_____

_____

9. List three examples of an abscess.

    a. _____

    b. _____

    c. _____

10. What are the signs of acute inflammation?

    a. _____

    b. _____

    c. _____

    d. _____

11. What happens when an ulcer is formed?

    a. _____

    b. _____

12. What are the characteristics of cellulitis?

_____

_____

_____

13. What are the causes of cellulitis?

    a. _____

    b. _____

    c. _____

14. How is cellulitis typically treated?

_____

_____

_____

15. What is the function of a scab?

_____

_____

_____

16. What is an opportunistic infection?

_____

_____

_____

17. Where do bacteria normally live?

    a. _____

    b. _____

    c. _____

    d. _____

    e. _____

18. What does the abbreviation MRSA stand for?

_____

19. List common infections caused by the bacterium *streptococcus*.

    a. _____

    b. _____

    c. _____

    d. _____

20. What immunizations are effective in preventing viral infections?

    a. _____

    b. _____

    c. _____

    d. _____

    e. _____

21. List four common fungal infections.

    a. _____

    b. _____

    c. _____

    d. _____

True / False

____ 1. Once an individual no longer has pain or drainage in an infection site, it is okay to stop taking the prescribed antibiotics.

____ 2. Good hand washing is the best preventive measure against the common cold.

CASE STUDY

Stephen, age 17, developed a rash and possible skin infection on his arms and torso. He has had a cold for a couple weeks and has also had an elevated temperature at times. He was not concerned about the cold but since he developed the rash with some draining vesicles, he has become very anxious about the problem. His mother made an appointment for him to see his primary care physician since she is worried that he has developed an infection along with the rash.

1. List some symptoms of infection.

_____

_____

2. What diagnostic tests might Stephen's physician use to determine if he has an infection. What type of infection might he have?

_____

_____

Common Diseases and Disorders of Body Systems

CHAPTER 5

Immune System Diseases and Disorders

Define Terms

Define the following terms:

1. allergy _____

2. streptococcal _____

3. prophylactic _____

4. bronchospasm _____

5. allergen _____

Matching

Match the following terms with the correct definition:

_____ 1. autoimmune	A. hives
_____ 2. antigen	B. RF
_____ 3. hemolytic	C. immunity against self
_____ 4. rheumatoid factor	D. destroys blood
_____ 5. urticaria	E. cell marker that causes a state of sensitivity to an antibody
	F. dry eyes

Match the following terms with the correct definition:

_____ 6. immunodeficiency	A. lack of immunity
_____ 7. ptosis	B. severe allergic reaction
_____ 8. cytoxic	C. cell killing
_____ 9. anaphylaxis	D. double vision
_____ 10. diplopia	E. immunity against self
	F. drooping eyelids

Identify Diagnostic Tests

Fill in the blank:

1. The most important test for diagnosing allergies is _____.

2. The test that indicates the formation of antibodies on the red blood cell is the _____.

3. Autoimmune disorders may be diagnosed utilizing _____ tests that measure for specific diseases.

4. Finding an antibody against the human immunodeficiency virus (HIV) is indicative of exposure to _____.

Condition Table

Complete the following table:

Condition and Definition	Signs and Symptoms	Diagnostic Tests	Treatment Plan
Hay fever			
Asthma			
Urticaria			
Anaphylaxis			
Contact Dermatitis			
Rheumatic Fever			
Rheumatoid Arthritis			
Myasthenia Gravis			
Lupus Erythematosus			
Scleroderma			
Blood Transfusion Reaction			
Organ Rejection			
AIDS			

Completion

Using the words in the list, complete the following statements:

acetylcholine	itching
anaphylaxis	lymphocytes
antigens	redness
diffuse	self-antigen
discoid	swelling
heat	T-cells
human immunodeficiency virus	thymus
hypersensitivity disorder	
inflammation	
isoimmune disorder	

1. _____ are the major cells of the immune system.

2. _____, _____, _____, and _____ are common inflammatory responses to allergic reactions.

3. The result of an overreaction of the immune system to an antigen is called a _____ _____.

4. _____ is a severe allergic response to an allergen.

5. Autoimmune disorders are hypersensitivities in which the body fails to recognize its own _____.

6. Rheumatoid arthritis begins with _____ of the synovial lining of a joint.

7. Myasthenia gravis disrupts the transmission of _____, which affects the nerve impulses going to the muscles.

8. The two types of lupus erythematosus include _____ and _____.

9. _____ refers to a hypersensitivity of one person to another person's tissue.

10. _____ on the red blood cells give each type of cell a special identify.

11. The cause of AIDS is a _____ _____ _____.

12. As the _____ gland decreases in size with aging, so does the number of _____.

Short Answer

Provide answers to the following:

1. What are the primary and secondary organs of the immune system?

   a. _____

   b. _____

   c. _____

   d. _____

   e. _____

   f. _____

2. List the cells of the immune system.

    a. _____

    b. _____

    c. _____

    d. _____

    e. _____

3. Name two types of immune responses.

    a. _____

    b. _____

4. List the different types of immunity and give an example of each type.

    a. _____

    b. _____

    c. _____

    d. _____

5. What is natural immunity?

    _____

    _____

    _____

6. What is the clinical problem associated with immune deficiency disorders?

    _____

    _____

    _____

7. What are the two main groups of diseases of the immune system?

    a. _____

    b. _____

8. List the signs and symptoms of allergies.

    a. _____

    b. _____

    c. _____

    d. _____

    e. _____

    f. _____

    g. _____

9. Define *status asthmaticus.*

    _____

    _____

10. What are the triggers for nonallergic asthma?

    a. _____

    b. _____

    c. _____

    d. _____

11. What substances commonly cause anaphylactic reactions?

    a. _____

    b. _____

    c. _____

    d. _____

    e. _____

    f. _____

    g. _____

    h. _____

    i. _____

    j. _____

    k. _____

    l. _____

12. What are the symptoms of food allergies?

    a. _____

    b. _____

    c. _____

13. What allergens are common causes of contact dermatitis?

    a. _____

    b. _____

    c. _____

    d. _____

    e. _____

    f. _____

    g. _____

14. What are autoimmune disorders?

    _____

    _____

    _____

15. List some examples of autoimmune disorders.

    a. _____

    b. _____

    c. _____

    d. _____

    e. _____

16. When does chronic organ rejection occur?

    _____

    _____

    _____

17. What is an immunodeficiency disorder?

    _____

    _____

    _____

18. How is immune deficiency acquired?

    a. _____

    b. _____

    c. _____

19. What disorders commonly lead to immunodeficiency?

    a. _____

    b. _____

    c. _____

    d. _____

20. List the four stages of HIV.

    a. _____

    b. _____

    c. _____

    d. _____

21. List the three primary ways HIV can be spread or transmitted.

    a. _____

    b. _____

    c. _____

True / False

_____ 1. Research is now being conducted to determine if altering adaptive immunity can reduce tumor growth and the spread of cancer.

_____ 2. The immune system is important in preserving the body's immunity by eliminating tumors that produce antigens.

_____ 3. Echinacea, vitamin C, and zinc have all been promoted as cold remedies.

_____ 4. The research consensus is that vitamin C and zinc are the best alternative medicines to use to prevent the common cold.

_____ 5. Research has shown that alternative therapies for food allergies are producing very positive effects for the people suffering from these allergies.

_____ 6. Most research related to AIDS has been done on women and children.

_____ 7. One strategy to prevent AIDS transmission is to be sure to use birth control pills when engaging in sexual intercourse.

_____ 8. A recommended strategy to prevent AIDS transmission is to refrain from having multiple sex partners or having sex with intravenous drug users.

CASE STUDY

Jason, age 10, was brought to the emergency room by his mother. He had been stung by a bee and was having some difficulty breathing. She thought he might be having an anaphylactic reaction.

1. What are the symptoms of a localized anaphylactic reaction?

_____

_____

2. What are the symptoms of a systemic anaphylactic reaction?

_____

_____

3. What is the treatment for an anaphylactic reaction?

_____

_____

_____

CHAPTER **6**

Musculoskeletal System Diseases and Disorders

Define Terms

Define the following terms:

1. fascia _____

2. interphalangeal _____

3. mineralization _____

4. radiologic _____

5. sciatica _____

6. tetany _____

7. tophi _____

Matching

Match the following terms with the correct definition:

_____ 1. transverse   A. star-like pattern

_____ 2. oblique   B. runs across at a 90-degree angle

_____ 3. spiral   C. twisted around the bone

_____ 4. stellate   D. within the trochanter of the femur

_____ 5. intertrochanteric   E. run in a transverse pattern

Match the following terms with the correct definition:

_____ 6. open fracture   A. more than two ends or fragments

_____ 7. simple fracture   B. bone is protruding through the skin

_____ 8. comminuted   C. incomplete fracture

_____ 9. stress fracture   D. no opening in the skin

_____ 10. greenstick   E. too much weight-bearing or pressure

Define Abbreviations

Define the following abbreviations:

1. CAT _____
2. CT _____
3. MRI _____
4. ORIF _____
5. RICE _____
6. LBP _____
7. TMJ _____
8. HNP _____

Identify Diagnostic Tests

Fill in the blanks with the correct terms:

1. The primary tool utilized to diagnose bone and joint disorders is _____.

2. Testing that provides more detail than basic radiologic examination includes _____ and _____.

3. A radiologic examination that provides detailed pictures that appear to cut the area of consideration into slices is _____.

4. A radiologic examination that utilizes a large magnet to make electromagnetic images is _____.

5. _____ studies include calcium, phosphorus, and alkaline phosphatase.

6. Muscle disorders are often evaluated by _____.

Condition Table

Complete the following table:

Condition and Definition	Signs and Symptoms	Diagnostic Tests	Treatment Plan
Scoliosis			
Osteoporosis			
Osteomyelitis			
Osteoarthritis			
Rheumatoid Arthritis			
Muscular Dystrophy			
Fracture			

Herniated Nucleus Pulposus			
Bursitis			
Carpal Tunnel Syndrome			
Plantar Faciitis			
Cruciate Ligament Tear			

Completion

Using the words in the list, complete the following statements:

kyphosis	scoliosis
lordosis	striated
myelogram	tophi
rickets	

1. Muscle that looks like stripes or bands is _____.

2. Small, whitish nodules are called _____.

3. _____ is a humped abnormal curvature of the thoracic spine.

4. Lateral curvature of the spine is called _____.

5. _____ is also called *swayback*.

6. A special X-ray after the injection of dye into the spinal cord to reveal compression of the spinal cord or spinal nerves is called a _____.

Short Answer

Provide answers to the following:

1. What is the difference between cortical bone and cancellous bone?

   _____

   _____

   _____

2. List the steps of bone repair.

   a. _____

   b. _____

   c. _____

   d. _____

   e. _____

3. What factors may affect the healing process?

   a. _____

   b. _____

   c. _____

   d. _____

   e. _____

4. Describe a joint.

   _____

   _____

   _____

5. How are joints classified?

   a. _____

   b. _____

6. List the major movements of the joints.

   a. _____

   b. _____

   c. _____

   d. _____

   e. _____

   f. _____

   g. _____

7. What are the functions of cartilage?

   a. _____

   b. _____

   c. _____

   d. _____

8. What are the functions of muscles?

   a. _____

   b. _____

9. What are tendons?

   _____

   _____

   _____

10. What are common signs and symptoms of bone and joint disease?

   a. _____

   b. _____

   c. _____

   d. _____

11. What are the primary tumors of the bone marrow?

    a. _____

    b. _____

12. What are the most common symptoms of the musculoskeletal system?

    a. _____

    b. _____

13. What are the causes of fractures?

    a. _____

    b. _____

14. Describe the following fractures:

    a. open _____

    b. closed or simple _____

    c. greenstick _____

    d. displaced _____

    e. nondisplaced _____

    f. comminuted _____

    g. compression _____

    h. impacted _____

    i. avulsion _____

    j. longitudinal _____

    k. transverse _____

    l. oblique _____

    m. spiral _____

    n. stellate _____

    o. intracapsular _____

    p. extracapsular _____

    q. intertrochanteric _____

    r. femoral neck/subcapital _____

15. How are fractures treated?

    a. _____

    b. _____

    c. _____

    d. _____

    e. _____

16. What is the benefit of traction when treating fractures?

    a. _____

    b. _____

    c. _____

17. What are two types of traction?

    a. _____

    b. _____

18. What are the complications of fractures?

    a. _____

    b. _____

    c. _____

    d. _____

19. What does the acronym RICE mean?

    R _____

    I _____

    C _____

    E _____

20. What happens to the musculoskeletal system as an individual ages?

    a. _____

    b. _____

    c. _____

    d. _____

    e. _____

    f. _____

True / False

_____ 1. The Korean preparation of *Gami-Honghwain* (HJ), which contains safflower seeds, has been tested for use in the treatment of bone diseases.

_____ 2. HJ has been found to be an excellent preparation to help bones heal faster.

_____ 3. Knuckle cracking causes arthritis in the joints.

_____ 4. If you have an injury that has not improved in 7–10 days, you should see a physician.

_____ 5. Application of ice on an injury slows bleeding and swelling by causing vasoconstriction.

_____ 6. Antioxidant supplements and aerobic training may help prevent bone loss in the elderly.

_____ 7. There is no benefit to using vitamins and aerobic training in the elderly to decrease bone loss.

_____ 8. Ice should be applied directly to the skin immediately after an injury.

CASE STUDY

George, age 28, is an avid jogger. He has had some difficulty with shin splints in the past, especially when he has not jogged for a few days and then restarts his exercise routine. He tripped yesterday while jogging and twisted his ankle. He is concerned that he might have sprained it.

1. What are the common symptoms of shin splints?

   _____

   _____

   _____

2. What is the treatment for shin splints?

   _____

   _____

   _____

3. What is a strain?

   _____

   _____

   _____

4. What are the symptoms of a strain?

   _____

   _____

   _____

5. If George has a strain, how should it be treated?

   _____

   _____

6. What is a sprain?

   _____

   _____

   _____

7. What are the symptoms of a sprain?

   _____

   _____

   _____

8. If George has a sprain, how should it be treated?

   _____

   _____

CHAPTER 7

Blood and Blood-Forming Organs Diseases and Disorders

Define Terms

Define the following terms:

1. anemia _____

2. ecchymosis _____

3. erythrocytopenia _____

4. hemarthrosis _____

5. hematemesis _____

6. hematuria _____

7. hemoglobin _____

8. leukocytosis _____

9. pallor _____

10. petechiae _____

11. syncope _____

12. thrombocytosis _____

Matching

Match the following terms with the correct definition:

_____ 1. aplastic anemia

_____ 2. pernicious anemia

_____ 3. hemolytic anemia

_____ 4. sickle cell anemia

_____ 5. hemorrhagic anemia

A. neoplasms of lymphoid tissue

B. failure of bone marrow to produce blood components

C. lack of intrinsic factor

D. acute loss of large amounts of blood

E. increased destruction of red blood cells

F. an inherited anemia

Match the following terms with the correct definition:

_____ 6. hemophilia

_____ 7. pancytopenia

_____ 8. mononucleosis

_____ 9. leukemia

_____ 10. lymphoma

A. decrease in the oxygen-carrying ability of the red blood cell

B. "blood lover," needs transfusions

C. "kissing disease"

D. abnormally high number of immature leukocytes

E. malignant neoplasm of blood-forming organs

F. decrease or absence of erythrocytes, leukocytes, and thrombocytes

Define Abbreviations

Define the following abbreviations:

1. RBC _____

2. CBC _____

3. WBC _____

4. HGB _____

5. HCT _____

Identify Diagnostic Tests

Fill in the blanks with the correct terms:

1. A common blood test that measures the number of RBCs, WBCs, and platelets is called a _____ .

2. A _____ _____ _____ is a test that provides a detailed count identifying the number of each type of leukocyte.

3. A microscopic examination that identifies the shape of the cells and platelets is a _____ _____.

4. The time it takes for a pricked earlobe to quit bleeding is a test called _____ _____.

5. A test performed by boring a needle into the bone of the iliac crest of the hip to obtain tissue for examination is a _____ _____ _____.

Condition Table

Complete the following table:

Condition and Definition	Signs and Symptoms	Diagnostic Tests	Treatment Plan
Anemia			
Polycythemia			
Leukemia			
Lymphoma			

Multiple Myeloma			
Hemophilia			
Thrombocytopenia			
Disseminated Intravascular Coagulation			
Mononucleosis			

Completion

Using the words in the list, complete the following sentences:

anemia	plasma proteins
hemarthrosis	polycythemia
hematemesis	Reed-Sternberg
hemolyzed	sickle
multiple myeloma	water
pancytopenia	

1. The plasma portion of the blood is composed of _____ and _____ _____.

2. _____ means low or decreased blood volume.

3. An elongated cell with abnormal hemoglobin is called a _____ cell.

4. _____ is an absence or decrease of erythrocytes, leukocytes, and thrombocytes.

5. Too many blood cells is called _____.

6. A _____ cell is present in the lymphatic tissue in Hodgkin's disease.

7. An excess of calcium may be found in the blood in _____.

8. _____ cells are ones which are broken down.

9. Vomiting blood is also called _____.

10. Bleeding into the joints is called _____.

Short Answer

Provide answers to the following:

1. What is the major function of the blood?

2. What is the role of leukocytes?

_____

_____

_____

3. Describe plasma.

_____

_____

_____

4. What is the function of erythrocytes?

_____

_____

_____

5. What happens to worn-out red blood cells?

a. _____

b. _____

6. What is the function of hemoglobin?

_____

_____

_____

7. What is the function of leukocytes?

_____

_____

_____

8. What is the indication of a white blood cell count greater than 11,000?

_____

_____

_____

9. Describe the composition of plasma.

_____

_____

_____

10. List the phases of blood coagulation.

a. _____

b. _____

c. _____

d. _____

11. List the four types of blood.

    a. _____

    b. _____

    c. _____

    d. _____

12. What is the difference between Rh-negative blood and Rh-positive blood?

    _____

    _____

    _____

13. List the blood-forming organs.

    a. _____

    b. _____

    c. _____

    d. _____

    e. _____

14. What are the common symptoms of erythrocytosis?

    a. _____

    b. _____

    c. _____

    d. _____

    e. _____

15. What happens when an individual has leukocytopenia?

    _____

    _____

    _____

16. What effect does leukocytosis have on the body?

    a. _____

    b. _____

17. What disorders or diseases may lead to anemia?

    a. _____

    b. _____

    c. _____

18. What are the causes of iron deficiency anemia?

    a. _____

    b. _____

19. What are the causes of folic acid deficiency anemia?

    a. _____

    b. _____

    c. _____

    d. _____

20. What ethnic group is affected by sickle cell anemia?

    _____

21. What is the theory to explain the development of sickle cell anemia?

    _____

    _____

    _____

22. Acute loss of large amounts of blood leads to what type of anemia?

    _____

    _____

    _____

    _____

23. What are the characteristics of aplastic anemia?

    _____

    _____

    _____

24. What are the causes of aplastic anemia?

    a. _____

    b. _____

    c. _____

    d. _____

25. What is the treatment for polycythemia?

    _____

    _____

    _____

26. What are the characteristics of leukemia?

    a. _____

    b. _____

27. What are the characteristics of Hodgkin's disease?

    a. _____

    b. _____

    c. _____

28. What is the cause of Hodgkin's disease?

    _____

    _____

    _____

29. What are the characteristics of thrombocytopenia?

    a. _____

    b. _____

    c. _____

    d. _____

    e. _____

    f. _____

30. When does disseminated intravascular coagulation occur?

    _____

    _____

    _____

31. What is the most common disorder of the blood in the older adult?

    _____

True / False

_____ 1. Most alternative therapies used to treat sickle cell disease are very effective according to the individuals who are using them.

_____ 2. According to the research noted in the chapter, prayer and spiritual healing are the most frequently used alternative treatments for sickle cell disease.

_____ 3. Recently the FDA approved using an iron chelator called deferasirox for sickle cell anemia.

_____ 4. CAT scans are now being used to detect iron overload in patients who have had multiple blood transfusions for sickle cell anemia.

↻ CASE STUDY

Cindy, age 47, recently had a routine check up with her physician recently. She went in a week before the appointment to have some lab work done. She said she has been feeling a little tired most days but she does not have an elevated temperature, sore throat, or cough. The physician ordered a CBC for her.

1. What does CBC mean? _____

2. What tests are performed when a CBC is ordered?

   _____

   _____

   _____

   _____

   _____

Cardiovascular System Diseases and Disorders

Define Terms

Define the following terms:

1. auscultation _____

2. cardiac palpitations _____

3. cyanosis _____

4. fibrillation _____

5. ischemia _____

6. murmur _____

7. perfusion _____

8. systolic _____

9. tachycardia _____

10. thrombus _____

Matching

Match the following diagnostic terms with the correct definition:

_____ 1. dyspnea

_____ 2. hemoglobin

_____ 3. arteriogram

_____ 4. ultrasound

_____ 5. angiogram

A. X-ray of an artery

B. carries the oxygen in the blood

C. X-ray of a vessel

D. use of sound waves for diagnostic purposes

E. a device used for listening to the heart and movement of blood in vessels

F. shortness of breath

Match the following diagnostic terms with the correct definition:

_____ 6. patency

_____ 7. Doppler

_____ 8. embolus

_____ 9. prothrombin time

_____ 10. cardiac catheterization

A. material floating in the blood

B. a device that magnifies the sound of blood flow

C. X-ray of an artery

D. invasive procedure used to sample the blood in the chambers of the heart to determine the oxygen content

E. blood test to monitor the anticoagulant drug level

F. openness

Define Abbreviations

Define the following abbreviations:

1. CVA _____

2. EKG or ECG _____

3. MI _____

4. CABG _____

5. CPR _____

6. TPA _____

7. CHF _____

8. DVT _____

Identify Diagnostic Tests

Match the following diagnostic tests with the correct description below:

A. cardiac catheterization

B. angiography

C. electrocardiogram

D. venography

E. arterial blood pressure

F. Doppler

G. creatinine phosphokinase

H. echocardiography

I. auscultation

____ 1. The process of using a stethoscope to listen to the heart

____ 2. A graph picture of heart activity

____ 3. An invasive procedure used to sample the blood in the chambers of the heart to determine the oxygen content and blood pressure in the heart's chambers

____ 4. A device to magnify sounds of the heart and vessels

____ 5. Measured by a sphygmomanometer

____ 6. A blood enzyme indicative of a heart attack

____ 7. A noninvasive ultrasound of the heart

Condition Table

Complete the following table:

Condition and Definition	Symptoms	Diagnostic Tests	Treatment Plan
Myocardial Infarction			
Hypertensive Heart Disease			
Congestive Heart Failure			

Cardiomyopathy			
Phlebitis			
Varicose Veins			
Hemmorrhage			
Shock			

Completion

Using the words in the list, complete the following statements:

arrhythmia	blood pressure	bradycardia
diastolic	dyspnea	embolus
fibrillation	palpitations	plaque
systolic	tachycardia	

1. The top or first recorded number in the blood pressure, caused by the contraction of the ventricle is the _____ blood pressure.

2. Difficult breathing is also known as _____.

3. _____ _____ is the level of pressure of the blood pushing against the walls of the vessels as it is delivered throughout the body.

4. Fatty, cholesterol deposits in blood vessels are called _____.

5. A blood clot that breaks loose and floats in the blood, possibly occluding or stopping blood flow is known as a(n) _____.

6. An irregular heart rhythm is called a(n) _____.

7. A wild, uncontrolled arrhythmia is called a(n) _____.

8. Another word for rapid heart rate is _____.

9. An abnormal heart rate that the individual can feel or is very aware of is called _____.

10. _____ is a slow heart rate.

11. The bottom number or lower number in the blood pressure is known as the _____ blood pressure.

Short Answer

Describe the following surgical procedures and when they are indicated:

1. Coronary artery bypass graft

_____

_____

_____

2. Endarterectomy

_____

_____

_____

3. Angioplasty

_____

_____

_____

4. Vein stripping

_____

_____

_____

5. Embolectomy/thrombectomy

_____

_____

_____

For each of the following, describe the condition, then list the symptoms and describe how the disease/disorder is diagnosed:

6. Aneurysm

_____

_____

_____

7. Arteriosclerosis/atherosclerosis

_____

_____

_____

8. Cerebrovascular accident

_____

_____

_____

9. Coronary artery disease

_____

_____

_____

10. Deep vein thrombosis

_____

_____

_____

11. Rheumatic heart disease

_____

_____

_____

_____

12. Peripheral vascular disease

_____

_____

_____

True / False

____ 1. Grape seed extract has been used as a remedy for reducing hypertension.

____ 2. Free radicals have been linked to damage in cell membranes.

____ 3. Antioxidants are ineffective in the presence of free radicals.

____ 4. Researchers are trying to develop drugs to lower high blood pressure without the side effects of medicines used today.

____ 5. To help lower the risk for cardiovascular disease, an individual should reduce salt intake.

____ 6. An individual needs to have his blood pressure checked routinely only if he has a cardiovascular disease such as hypertension.

CASE STUDY

Evelyn, age 57, is a very active lady in the community. She volunteers at the hospital and also at her church. Lately she had been feeling weak, short of breath, and has had some minor chest and leg pains. She has also been having headaches. She knows she is 20 pounds overweight but still has been able to get around fine without any significant trouble. Her physician told her that she has hypertension and some atherosclerosis. She was surprised to hear this because, until recently, she has felt fine. She asked him why she has these problems at this time. He stated some of this is probably due to heredity but some is related to her lifestyle.

1. The genetic and environmental risk factors contributing to primary hypertension are _____, _____, _____, _____, _____, _____, and _____.

2. The controllable factors contributing to atherosclerosis are _____, _____, _____, _____, _____, _____, and _____.

3. The noncontrollable factors contributing to atherosclerosis are _____, _____, _____, and _____.

Respiratory System Diseases and Disorders

Define Terms

Define the following terms:

1. apnea _____

_____

2. bronchiectasis _____

_____

3. clubbing _____

_____

4. dyspnea _____

_____

5. hemoptysis _____

_____

6. cyanosis _____

_____

7. sputum _____

_____

8. hypoxia _____

_____

9. orthopnea _____

_____

10. tachypnea _____

_____

Matching

Match the disease with the correct identifier:

_____ 1. hay fever

_____ 2. pharyngitis

_____ 3. chronic bronchitis

_____ 4. pulmonary abscess

_____ 5. tuberculosis

A. sore throat

B. "shock lung"

C. lung abscess

D. "consumption"

E. allergic rhinitis

F. "smoker's cough"

Match the following terms with the correct identifier:

____ 6. adult respiratory distress syndrome

____ 7. pleural effusion

____ 8. coccidioidomycosis

____ 9. Legionnaire's disease

____ 10. laryngitis

A. "desert fever"

B. hydrothorax

C. "consumption"

D. "shock lung"

E. bacterial pneumonia

F. hoarseness

Define Abbreviations

Define the following abbreviations:

1. ABG _____

2. PE _____

3. URI _____

4. TB _____

5. CO_2 _____

6. PFT _____

7. COPD _____

Identify Diagnostic Tests

Match the test with the correct identifier:

A. auscultation

B. chest roentgenogram

C. bronchoscopy

D. arterial blood gases

E. oxygen saturation

F. pulmonary function tests

G. spirometer

____ 1. A group of tests measuring volume and flow of air into the lungs

____ 2. A procedure to look into the lungs

____ 3. The primary or major diagnostic tool

____ 4. A measurement of oxygen and carbon dioxide in the blood

____ 5. A measurement or metered tool to measure lung function

Condition Table

Complete the following table:

Condition and Definition	Symptoms	How Diagnosed	Treatment
Common Cold			
Hay Fever			

Sinusitis			
Pharyngitis			
Acute Bronchitis			
Influenza			
Chronic Obstructive Lung Disease			
Pneumonia			
Tuberculosis			
Pleurisy			
Pulmonary Embolism			
Legionnaire's Disease			
Pneumothorax			

Completion

Use the words in the list to complete the following statements:

orthopnea	rales
rhinorrhea	hypoxia
hemoptysis	dyspnea
antipyretics	apnea
clubbing	analgesics

1. _____ is when the individual is unable to breathe unless the individual is in a sitting position.

2. Musical sounds heard when listening to the lungs are called _____.

3. A runny nose is also called _____.

4. The medical term for low oxygen in the blood is _____.

5. The medical term for coughing up blood is _____.

6. Bad, painful, or difficult breathing is called _____.

7. Medications used to reduce fevers are called _____.

8. Absence of respirations is known as _____.

9. _____ is due to poor distal circulation and oxygenation.

10. Pain relievers are called _____.

Use the words in the list to complete the following statements:

cyanosis	tachypnea
rhonchi	thoracentesis
sputum	wheezing
alveoli	productive cough
bronchoscopy	biopsy

11. A bluish color to the skin is called _____.

12. Rapid breathing is known as _____.

13. Dry, rattling sounds when listening to the lungs is called _____.

14. The surgical puncture of the thorax is known as _____.

15. _____ is fluids or secretions coughed up from the lungs.

16. _____ is high-pitched whistling sounds caused by partial obstruction of the lungs.

17. The grape-like clusters of air sacs at the distal end of the terminal bronchioles are known as _____.

18. A(n) _____ _____ is one in which there is sputum of excessive mucus.

19. The visual examination of the bronchi is called _____.

20. Removing tissue for examination under the microscope is known as a(n) _____.

Use the words in the list to complete the following statements:

hay fever	sinusitis
sore throat	laryngitis
influenza	chronic obstructive pulmonary disease
atelectasis	pneumonia
tuberculosis	lung cancer

21. Allergic rhinitis is commonly known as _____.

22. _____ is inflammation of the mucous membrane lining of the sinuses.

23. Pharyngitis is commonly known as a(n) _____ _____.

24. Inflammation of the vocal cords and larynx is called _____.

25. A highly contagious respiratory infection characterized by sudden onset of fever, chills, headache, and back pain is called _____.

26. A group of diseases characterized by the inability to get air in and out of the lungs is known as _____ _____ _____ _____.

27. Collapse or airless state of part or the entire lung is called _____.

28. Inflammation of the lung is called _____.

29. _____ was formerly called consumption.

30. _____ _____ is the leading cause of cancer deaths in the United States.

Use the words in the list to complete the following statements:

pleurisy	pneumothorax
thoracentesis	pleural effusion
pulmonary embolus	histoplasmosis/coccidioidomycosis
smoking	respiratory infection
upper respiratory infections	rhinovirus

31. Inflammation of the membranes covering the lung is called _____.

32. Collection of air in the pleural space is called _____.

33. _____ is a procedure done in order to withdraw air and insert a chest tube to assist in reexpanding the lung.

34. A collection of fluid in the chest is known as _____.

35. A clot that commonly develops in the legs, breaks off, and gets stuck in the pulmonary artery is called a(n) _____ _____.

36. _____ is an example of a fungal disease of the lung.

37. _____ is the most preventable risk factor for developing lung cancer.

38. The type of infection that accounts for approximately 80 percent of all infections is called _____ _____.

39. The most common cause for lost days of work for adults is _____ _____ _____.

40. The name of the virus responsible for upper respiratory infections is _____.

Short Answer

Provide answers to the following:

1. Describe mechanical ventilation.

_____

_____

_____

2. Describe influenza immunization.

_____

_____

_____

3. Describe a surgical resection of the lung.

_____

_____

_____

4. Describe a salt-water gargle.

_____

_____

_____

True / False

____ 1. Smoking is the main cause of preventable death in the U.S.

____ 2. Smoking can cause an increased heart rate.

____ 3. Smoking is strongly linked to kidney disease and failure.

_____ 4. The QuantiFERON-TB (QFT) test is recommended by the CDC for TB testing.

_____ 5. The use of vitamin preparations and other herbal remedies for treating pulmonary disorders is increasing but the value of these treatments has not been well established.

_____ 6. Some research studies have reported that a form of tocopherol, called α-tocopherol, found in many dietary supplements, is just as effective for allergic rhinitis as y-tocopherol, which is the primary form of dietary vitamin E.

CASE STUDY

Joe, age 72, has been diagnosed with pleural effusion. He is having difficulty breathing. The physician said he would need a thoracentesis to relieve the pressure and help his breathing pattern improve.

Describe a thoracentesis procedure.

_____

_____

_____

Lymphatic System Diseases and Disorders

Define Terms

Define the following terms:

1. lymph _____

    _____

2. lymphocytes _____

    _____

3. lymphocytosis _____

    _____

4. lymphocytopenia _____

    _____

5. lymphedema _____

    _____

Define Terms

Definite the following word forms:

1. lymph _____
2. angio _____
3. adeno _____
4. opathy _____
5. graphy _____
6. itis _____
7. edema _____
8. cyto _____
9. osis _____
10. penia _____

Condition Table

Complete the following table:

Condition and Definition	Symptoms	Diagnostic Tests	Treatment Plan
Lymphoma			
Kawasaki Disease			
Lymphedema			
Lymphadenitis			

Completion

Use the words in the list to complete the following statements:

Kawasaki disease	lymphocytes
lymph	lymphocytopenia
lymphadenitis	lymphocytosis
lymphadenopathy	lymphomas
lymphangiography	mononucleosis
lymphangiopathy	Reed-Sternberg (RS)
lymphedema	vessels, ducts, nodes

1. Inflammation of the lymph gland and/or nodes is known as _____.

2. Neoplasms that affect lymphoid tissue are called _____.

3. _____ is fluid of the lymph system.

4. White blood cells created in the lymphatic system are called _____.

5. Inflammation of the lymph glands is called _____.

6. An X-ray of the lymph vessels is called _____.

7. A collection of lymph fluid usually in the extremities is called _____.

8. Disease of the lymph vessels is called _____.

9. _____ _____ is also called mucocutaneous lymph node syndrome.

10. _____ is also called the "kissing disease."

11. Decreased lymphocytes is known medically as _____.

12. Increased lymphocytes are medically called _____.

13. Disease of the lymph glands is called _____.

14. The _____ _____ cell confirms the diagnosis of Hodgkin's disease.

15. The lymphatic system includes the _____, _____, and _____.

Short Answer

Provide answers to the following:

1. List the components of the lymph system.

   _____

   _____

   _____

2. What is the goal of the lymphatic system?

   _____

   _____

   _____

3. What is the job of the lymphatic system?

   _____

   _____

   _____

4. List the common signs and symptoms of the lymphatic system.

   a. _____

   b. _____

   c. _____

   d. _____

5. What diagnostic tests are performed in order to confirm a diagnosis of the lymph system?

   a. _____

   b. _____

   c. _____

   d. _____

   e. _____

   f. _____

True / False

_____ 1. In October 2006, the Food and Drug Administration (FDA) approved the use of a new alternative treatment for post–breast cancer lymphedema.

_____ 2. The Riancorp LTU-904 Laser Therapy Unit is the only laser device approved by the FDA for lymphedema treatment.

_____ 3. New research is looking at weight reduction as a treatment for women who have lymphedema after a mastectomy.

_____ 4. The Food and Drug Administration (FDA) approved the use of a new laser therapy device for the treatment of any type of lymphedema.

_____ 5. Weight reduction programs are highly recommended for women with lymphedema after a mastectomy.

CASE STUDY

Janet, age 19, is a college student. She is not eating or sleeping well, and she recently developed a sore throat. She visited the college health center and was diagnosed with mononucleosis.

1. Describe mononucleosis.

   _____

2. What treatment should she expect?

   _____

Digestive System Diseases and Disorders

Define Terms

Define the following terms:

1. hematochezia _____

_____

2. diarrhea _____

_____

3. jejunum _____

_____

4. achlorhydria _____

_____

5. defecate _____

_____

6. epigastric _____

_____

7. vermiform _____

_____

8. ileus _____

_____

9. diverticula _____

_____

10. asymptomatic _____

_____

Matching

Match the following terms with the correct definition:

____ 1. an abnormal opening in a tissue or organ

____ 2. inflammation of the peritoneum

____ 3. contraction of muscles along the gastrointestinal tract to move food

____ 4. vomiting blood

____ 5. tarry, dark stool

A. melena

B. peritonitis

C. peristalsis

D. intrinsic factor

E. hematemesis

F. perforation

Match the following terms with the correct definition:

_____ 6. inflammation of the gums

_____ 7. parts of tissue that cling to the surface of adjoining organs as scar tissue

_____ 8. hidden

_____ 9. symptoms flare up or become worse

_____ 10. general ill feeling

A. occult

B. dental plaque

C. malaise

D. adhesions

E. exacerbation

F. gingivitis

Match the following terms with the correct definition:

_____ 11. varicose veins in the rectum

_____ 12. inflammation of the appendix

_____ 13. outpouching of the small intestine and peritoneum into the groin area

_____ 14. inflammation of tissue at the lower end of the esophagus

_____ 15. inflammation of the stomach and intestine

A. gastroenteritis

B. inguinal hernia

C. hemorrhoids

D. gastritis

E. appendicitis

F. reflux esophagitis

Define Abbreviations

Define the following abbreviations:

1. NPO _____

2. UGI _____

3. EGD _____

4. O&P _____

5. IBD _____

6. IBS _____

Identify Diagnostic Tests

Define the following diagnostic tests:

1. colonoscopy _____

2. sigmoidoscopy _____

3. occult blood _____

4. ova and parasites _____

5. upper GI series _____

6. barium enema _____

7. gastroscopy _____

8. esophagogastroduodenoscopy _____

9. stool culture _____

10. biopsy _____

Condition Table

Complete the following table:

Condition and Definition	Symptoms	Diagnostic Tests	Treatment Plan
Appendicitis			
Reflux Esophagitis			
Pharyngitis			
Crohn's Disease			
Esophageal Varices			
Gastritis			
Peptic Ulcer			
Dysentery			
Colorectal Cancer			
Hemorrhoids			
Hernias Inguinal			
Diverticulitis/Diverticulosis			
Gastroenteritis			

Completion

Use the words in the list to complete the following statements:

duodenum, jejunum, and ileum body

cecum intrinsic factor   pylorus

endoscopy   diarrhea

constipation   periodontal disease

sore throat   gingivitis

peristalsis   reflux esophagitis

fundus

1. The three sections of the small intestine are the _____, _____, and _____.

2. Movement of food from the pharynx to the stomach is called _____.

3. The first section of the colon is called the _____.

4. The three parts of the stomach are the _____, _____, and _____.

5. The substance necessary for the absorption of vitamin B is called the _____ _____.

6. The condition caused by hard, dry stool is called _____.

7. Loose, watery stools are called _____.

8. The procedure allowing a physician to look directly into the digestive organs is called _____.

9. The main reason for tooth loss is _____ _____.

10. Inflammation of the gums is called _____.

11. The common name for pharyngitis is _____ _____.

12. The backflow of stomach acids through the cardiac sphincter upward into the esophagus is called _____ _____.

Use the words in the list to complete the following statements:

achlorhydria   strangulation

asymptomatic   sprue or celiac disease

pernicious anemia   melena

Crohn's disease   ileus

diverticulitis   hiatal hernia

esophageal varices   hemorrhoids

gastritis

13. A _____ _____ is the sliding of part of the stomach into the chest cavity.

14. _____ _____ are enlargements of the veins of the esophagus.

15. Inflammation of the stomach is called _____.

16. _____ _____ is the result of the loss of intrinsic factor.

17. Absence of symptoms is also known as _____.

18. _____ is dark, tarry stools.

19. The absence of hydrochloric acid is called _____.

20. Absence of peristalsis is called _____.

21. Varicose veins of the rectum are called _____.

22. Parts of the intestine that are herniated and become twisted, thus cutting off the blood supply to the organ are called a _____.

23. Inflammatory bowel syndrome is also called _____ _____.

24. The inflammation of the diverticula is called _____.

25. The condition that causes an individual to be sensitive to gluten proteins is called
_____ _____.

Short Answer

Provide answers to the following:

1. What are the purposes of the digestive system?

_____

_____

2. Trace a piece of food from the mouth to the anus.

_____

_____

3. What are the most common signs and symptoms of gastrointestinal disorders?

_____

_____

4. List some causes of constipation.

_____

_____

5. List some causes of diarrhea.

_____

_____

6. List some effects of aging on the gastrointestinal system.

_____

_____

True / False

____ 1. A low-fiber diet is essential for good GI function.

____ 2. Continued use of laxative preparations can disrupt the normal GT function.

____ 3. A strep throat is best diagnosed by inspection.

____ 4. Antibiotics should be taken as prescribed until all capsules are gone.

____ 5. Colon cancer is most common before age 40.

____ 6. Most microorganisms ingested are destroyed by acid in the stomach.

____ 7. Good hand washing is a preventive strategy for avoiding food poisoning.

____ 8. The juice of the Japanese apricot (prunus mume) has been studied as a treatment for *Helicobacter pylori* bacteria, which cause stomach ulcers.

____ 9. The effects of the banaba leaves in preventing diabetes have been confirmed in some studies.

____ 10. A unique test has been developed that examines the stomach without the tubes (gastroscope or EGD) that are usually used for this visualization.

CASE STUDY

Sue is a 36-year-old registered nurse who has been experiencing pain in the epigastric area after eating spicy foods. She has been complaining of the symptoms for the past few weeks.

1. What disease might she be diagnosed with?

_____

2. How would the diagnosis be made?

_____

3. How would this disease be treated?

_____

_____

_____

_____

_____

_____

_____

CHAPTER 12

Liver, Gallbladder, and Pancreatic Diseases and Disorders

Define Terms

Define the following terms:

1. abdominocentesis _____

2. ascites _____

3. cholecystectomy _____

4. esophageal varices _____

5. hematemesis _____

6. hepatomegaly _____

7. jaundice _____

8. splenomegaly _____

Matching

Match the following terms with the correct definition:

____ 1. a yellow skin color related to bile pigments in the blood

____ 2. occurring suddenly, rapidly and intensely

____ 3. digestion of self or one's own cells

____ 4. fluid in the abdomen

____ 5. a serious condition due to alcohol withdrawal

A. jaundice

B. ascites

C. autodigestion

D. delirium tremens

E. fulminant

F. gynecomastia

Identify Diagnostic Tests

Match the following diagnostic tests with the correct definition:

____ 1. cholecystogram

____ 2. amylase

____ 3. needle biopsy

____ 4. alkaline phosphatase

____ 5. albumin

____ 6. cholangiogram

____ 7. abdominocentesis

____ 8. lithotripsy

____ 9. liver function tests

____ 10. ultrasound

A. blood protein

B. X-ray of the gallbladder

C. evaluates the liver, gallbladder, and pancreas for size, shape, and position

D. surgical puncture of abdomen

E. measures pancreatic function

F. enzyme

G. sound waves used to break up stones

H. measures levels of bilirubin, albumin, and alkaline phosphatase

I. X-ray of the vessels of the gallbladder

J. most reliable test for diagnosis of cancer, chronic hepatitis, and cirrhosis

Condition Table

Complete the following table:

Condition and Definition	Symptoms	Diagnostic Tests	Treatment Plan
Cirrhosis			
Hepatitis B			
Cholecystitis			
Cholelithiasis			
Pancreatitis			

Completion

Using the words in the list, complete the following statements:

autodigestion   jaundice

cholelithiasis   hyperbilirubinemia

lithotripsy   emesis

ascites   hematemesis

1. Eating one's self is called _____ _____.

2. The yellowish discoloration of the skin is known as _____.

3. Gallstones are medically called _____.

4. Excessive bilirubin in the blood is called _____.

5. The use of sound waves to break up gallstones is called _____.

6. Vomiting is also called _____.

7. _____ is the accumulation of fluid in the abdomen.

8. Vomiting blood is also called _____.

Using the words in the list, complete the following statements:

abdominocentesis	spider angiomas
cholangiogram	pancreatitis
cholecystitis	liver
cholecystogram	hepatomegaly
hepatitis	fulminant

9. _____ is an enlarged liver.

10. Small dilated blood vessels on the face and chest are called _____ _____.

11. _____ is puncture of the abdomen.

12. A _____ is an X-ray of the gallbladder.

13. Inflammation of the liver is commonly called _____.

14. _____ is when something occurs suddenly and with great intensity.

15. The _____ is the largest solid organ of the body.

16. Inflammation of the gallbladder is called _____.

17. X-ray of the vessels of the gallbladder is called _____.

Short Answer

Please provide answers to the following:

1. Describe the functions of the liver.

   _____

   _____

   _____

2. Identify two signs and symptoms of liver problems.

   _____

   _____

3. Describe bile and its function.

   _____

   _____

4. The pancreas is both an endocrine and exocrine gland. What does this mean?

   _____

   _____

   _____

5. What are the secretions of the pancreas?

   _____

   _____

6. Older adults may be at risk for pancreatitis if what factors are present?

   _____

   _____

True / False

_____ 1. Interferon is a treatment strategy for HBV.

_____ 2. RNA interference (RNAi) may be a treatment strategy used in the future for HBV.

_____ 3. Herbal medicines are never harmful to the liver.

_____ 4. Statins mixed with herbal preparations are a good remedy for liver disease.

CASE STUDY

Jean is 45 years old and 50 pounds overweight. For the past 3 weeks, Jean has been experiencing severe right upper gastric pain after eating.

1. What disease might Jean have?

_____

_____

2. What predisposing factors does she have?

_____

_____

3. What symptoms does she have to support your diagnosis?

_____

_____

4. How would your diagnosis be confirmed?

_____

_____

5. What treatment would be done?

_____

_____

_____

CHAPTER 13

Urinary System Diseases and Disorders

Define Terms

Define the following terms:

1. anuria _____

2. catheterization _____

3. cystoscopy _____

4. dysuria _____

5. hematuria _____

6. nephrectomy _____

7. nocturia _____

8. uremia _____

9. pyuria _____

10. suprapubic catheter _____

Matching Terms

Match the following terms with the correct definition:

A. hydronephrosis	D. glomerulonephritis
B. urinary tract infection	E. cystitis
C. renal calculi	F. dysuria

_____ 1. collection of urine in the renal pelvis due to obstruction

_____ 2. any infection of the urinary system

_____ 3. kidney stones

_____ 4. inflammation of the bladder

_____ 5. painful urination

Match the following terms with the correct definition:

A. pyelonephritis   D. uremia

B. renal failure   E. urethritis

C. polycystic disease   F. nephrectomy

_____ 6. multiple grape-like cysts

_____ 7. failure of the kidneys to perform the function of cleansing the blood of waste products

_____ 8. urine waste in the blood

_____ 9. inflammation of the urethra

_____ 10. excision of a kidney

Define Abbreviations

Define the following abbreviations:

1. KUB _____

2. TUR _____

3. IVP _____

4. BUN _____

5. C&S _____

6. UTI _____

Identify Diagnostic Tests

Match the following diagnostic tests with the correct definition:

_____ 1. clean catch

_____ 2. urine C&S

_____ 3. needle biopsy

_____ 4. blood urea nitrogen

_____ 5. creatinine clearance

_____ 6. urinalysis

_____ 7. KUB

_____ 8. lithotripsy

_____ 9. catheterization

_____ 10. cystoscopy

A. the most common test to diagnose urinary system diseases

B. X-ray exam of kidney, ureters, bladder

C. obtaining clean urine for culture

D. breaking up kidney stones

E. a blood test to measure kidney function

F. lab test used if urine shows abnormal WBC or bacteria

G. protein waste in the blood

H. obtaining a small piece of tissue to determine the presence of disease

I. sterile procedure of placing a tube in the bladder

J. looking into the bladder

Condition Table

Complete the following table:

Condition and Definition	Signs and Symptoms	Diagnostic Tests	Treatment Plan
Polycystic Disease			
Renal Failure			
Glomerulonephritis			
Cystitis			
Pyelonephritis			
Transitional Cell Carcinoma of the Bladder			
Hydronephrosis			

Completion

Using the words in the list, complete the following statements:

anuria	nocturia
cystitis	oliguria
cystoscopy	pyretic
dysuria	pyuria
hematuria	renal calculi
incontinence	urgency

1. Inflammation of the bladder is called _____.

2. Another term for fever is _____.

3. Kidney stones are also called _____ _____.

4. _____ is blood in the urine.

5. The need to urinate "right now" is called _____.

6. _____ is loss of control of urine.

7. The need to urinate at night is called _____.

8. Bad, painful, or difficult urination is called _____.

9. Scant urine production is called _____.

10. Visual examination of the bladder is called _____.

11. Absence of urine is called _____.

12. Pus in the urine is called _____.

Short Answer

Provide answers to the following:

1. Describe the anatomy of the urinary system.

   _____

   _____

   _____

2. What signs and symptoms are commonly seen in the urinary system disorders?

   _____

   _____

3. What is the function of the kidney?

   _____

   _____

   _____

4. Describe urine.

   _____

   _____

True / False

_____   1. Limiting fluid intake might prevent recurring urinary tract infections.

_____   2. Drinking cranberry juice is recommended to raise the pH of the urine to prevent infections.

_____   3. Some herbal medicines have been linked to bladder cancer.

_____   4. *Longdan Xieganwan* is a Chinese herbal preparation used for liver enhancement.

_____   5. Probiotic bacteria are used to treat several human disorders.

_____   6. Probiotics are viruses that supplement the GI tract to inactivate harmful bacteria.

_____   7. Supplements of probiotics are normally found in the GI tract.

_____   8. The probiotics most commonly used in medicine today are strains of *Lactobacillus* and *Bifidobacterium*.

CASE STUDY

Annabelle is a 23-year-old female who just got married. She woke up this morning with urgency, frequency, and burning.

1. What might be her medical problem?

   _____

2. What is the rationale for your answer?

   _____

   _____

3. What is the treatment for the problem?

   _____

   _____

   _____

Endocrine System Diseases and Disorders

Define Terms

Define the following terms:

1. adenoma _____

_____

2. androgen _____

_____

3. glucagon _____

_____

4. hirsutism _____

_____

5. Islets of Langerhans _____

_____

6. polyuria _____

_____

7. precocious _____

_____

8. striae _____

_____

9. tetany _____

_____

10. vasopressin _____

_____

Matching

Match the following terms with the correct definition:

____ 1. hyperpituitarism

____ 2. type 1 diabetes

____ 3. cretinism

____ 4. Graves' disease

____ 5. diabetes insipidus

A. formerly known as juvenile onset diabetes

B. decrease in the release of vasopressin

C. abnormal increase in the activity of the pituitary gland

D. hypothyroidism in infants and children

E. formerly known as adult onset diabetes

F. hyperthyroidism caused by an autoimmune disorder

Match the following terms with the correct definition:

____ 6. goiter

____ 7. Cushing's syndrome

____ 8. polydipsia

____ 9. Addison's disease

____ 10. type 2 diabetes

A. enlargement of the thyroid gland due to inadequate dietary iodine

B. formerly known as adult onset diabetes

C. overproduction of cortisone

D. overproduction of aldosterone

E. hypoadrenalism

F. excessive thirst or drinking

Define Abbreviations

Match the following abbreviations with the correct definition:

____ 1. TSH

____ 2. FSH

____ 3. GH

____ 4. ADH

____ 5. MSH

____ 6. ACTH

____ 7. LH

____ 8. ICSH

____ 9. IDDM

____ 10. STH

A. somatropic hormone

B. antidiuretic hormone

C. non-insulin-dependent diabetes mellitus

D. follicle-stimulating hormone

E. growth hormone

F. interstitial cell-stimulating hormone

G. adrenocorticotropin hormone

H. insulin-dependent diabetes mellitus

I. thyroid stimulating hormone

J. lutenizing hormone

K. melanocyte stimulating hormone

Identify Diagnostic Tests

Mark an "X" in front of basic diagnostic test utilized to diagnose endocrine disorders:

A. ____ CT

B. ____ MRI

C. ____ EKG

D. ____ Physical examination

E. ____ Blood tests

F. ____ EGD

G. ____ Colonoscopy

H. ____ Upper GI

Define Word Forms

Define the following word forms:

1. **dipsia** _____

_____

2. **poly** _____

_____

3. **anti** _____

_____

4. **uri** _____

_____

5. **oma** _____

_____

6. **glyc** _____

_____

7. **phagia** _____

_____

8. **adeno** _____

_____

9. **hyper** _____

_____

10. **hypo** _____

_____

Condition Table

Complete the following table:

Condition and Definition	Signs and Symptoms	Diagnostic Tests	Treatment Plan
Goiter			
Diabetes Mellitus			
Diabetes Insipidus			
Giantism			
Addison's Disease			
Hypothyroidism			
Hypogonadism			
Conn's Disease			
Hyperparathyroidism			

Completion

Use the words in the list to complete the following statements:

growth hormone	gigantism
dwarfism	diabetes insipidus
thyroxine	Graves' disease
thyroid storm	goiter
cretinism	hypoparathyroidism

1. _____ _____ promotes the growth and development of all body tissues.

2. Hyperpituitarism occurring before puberty is known as _____.

3. Hypopituitarism results in _____.

4. A decrease in the release of vasopressin results in _____.

5. The hormone _____ regulates metabolism.

6. Hyperthyroidism caused by an autoimmune condition is also known as _____.

7. _____ _____ is a life-threatening exacerbation of all symptoms of hyperthyroidism.

8. An enlargement of the thyroid gland due to inadequate dietary iodine is called _____.

9. Hypothyroidism in children is called _____.

10. Low blood calcium levels result in _____.

Use the words in the list to complete the following statements:

Addison's disease	Cushing's disease
diabetic coma	gestational diabetes
hypogonadism	insulin and glucagon
insulin shock	ketoacidosis
ketones	polydipsia, polyphagia, polyuria

11. _____ _____ is due to an overproduction of cortisol.

12. Undersecretion of hormones produced by the adrenal cortex is called _____.

13. The two hormones secreted by the pancreas are _____ and _____.

14. When cells burn fats and proteins for energy, they produce a waste product called _____.

15. The condition of having ketones in the blood, breath, and urine is called _____.

16. Three symptoms of diabetes mellitus include _____, _____, and _____.

17. A condition that comes on rapidly as a result of too much insulin is called _____ _____.

18. _____ _____ is the result of not administering enough insulin or taking in too many carbohydrates in the diet.

19. _____ _____ is a result of pregnancy.

20. Decreased production of sex hormones results in _____.

Short Answer

Provide answers to the following:

1. Describe the components of the endocrine system and their location.

   _____

   _____

   _____

2. List some common signs and symptoms of endocrine system disorders.

   _____

   _____

   _____

3. List the endocrine glands and their hormones.

   _____

   _____

   _____

   _____

   _____

   _____

   _____

4. List the symptoms of insulin shock.

   _____

   _____

5. List the symptoms of diabetic coma.

   _____

   _____

True / False

_____ 1. Anabolic steroids are synthetic derivatives of testosterone that have anabolic (tissue-building) effects.

_____ 2. The use of steroids to enhance athletic performance is not harmful if they are not used for a long period of time.

_____ 3. Individuals taking steroids should be on a well-balanced diet, including adequate proteins and carbohydrates.

_____ 4. A link has been found between vitamin D deficiency and the body's ability to metabolize glucose and insulin.

_____ 5. Although the relationship of vitamin D to insulin and glucose metabolism is still being investigated, in the future, vitamin D may be given to persons who are deficient to help prevent diabetes insipidus.

_____ 6. Complementary and alternative therapies are only used to treat type 1 diabetes.

_____ 7. *Clerodendrum capitatum* (CC) is a traditional African therapy for type 2 diabetes.

_____ 8. An individual should not use alternative medicines to treat diabetes mellitus without informing the primary care physician.

CASE STUDY

Lydia is a 50-year-old businesswoman who has noticed a slight enlargement in her neck. Her mother had a goiter at about the same age Lydia is now, so she is concerned that she may also have a goiter. She knows a goiter merely means enlargement of the thyroid gland.

What symptoms might Lydia exhibit if the goiter is due to hyperthyroidism?

_____

_____

_____

Nervous System Diseases and Disorders

Define Terms

Define the following terms:

1. intractable _____
   _____

2. paraesthesia _____
   _____

3. quadriplegia _____
   _____

4. cephalalgia _____
   _____

5. sleep apnea _____
   _____

6. amnesia _____
   _____

7. hypothermia _____
   _____

8. insomnia _____
   _____

9. seizure _____
   _____

10. hydrophobia _____
    _____

Matching Terms

Match the following terms with the correct definition:

1. nuchal rigidity

2. transient ischemic attacks

3. spinal stenosis

4. craniotomy

5. paraplegia

A. sudden, mild "mini strokes"

B. loss of movement in both legs

C. neck stiffness

D. narrowing of nerve root openings

E. loss of movement in all extremities

F. cutting into the skull

Match the following terms with the correct definition:

6. aura

7. dementia

8. endarterectomy

9. decompression

10. obstructive apnea

A. loss of mental ability

B. release pressure off the spinal cord

C. cleaning plaque out of an artery

D. fear of water

E. not breathing related to nasal blocking

F. sensation that precedes an event

Define Abbreviations

Define the following abbreviations:

1. **CSF** _____

   _____

2. **TIA** _____

   _____

3. **CVA** _____

   _____

4. **HNP** _____

   _____

5. **EEG** _____

   _____

Identify Diagnostic Tests

Define the following diagnostic tests:

1. spinal tap/lumbar puncture _____

   _____

2. electroencephalogram _____

   _____

3. motor testing _____

   _____

4. sensory testing _____

_____

5. mental or cognitive testing _____

_____

6. cerebrospinal fluid analysis _____

_____

7. myelogram _____

_____

8. angiograms _____

_____

Condition Table

Complete the following table:

Condition and Definition	Signs and Symptoms	Diagnostic Tests	Treatment Plan
Parkinson's Disease			
Concussion/Contusion			
Subdural Hematoma			
Meningitis			
Encephalitis			
Shingles			
Cerebrovascular Accident			
Transient Ischemic Attacks			
Headaches			
Epilepsy			
Bell's Palsy			
Alzheimer's Disease			
Sleep Apnea			

Completion

Use the words in the list to complete the following statements:

cephalalgia   convulsions

intractable   transient ischemic attacks

sleep apnea   insomnia

concussion   amnesia

craniotomy   hydrophobia

1. _____ is another name for headaches.

2. Abnormal muscle contractions are known as _____.

3. _____ means difficult to stop or control.

4. _____ _____ _____ are also called "mini strokes."

5. _____ _____ means without sleep.

6. The inability to fall or stay asleep is called _____.

7. A blow to the head by an object, fall, or other trauma is known as a(n) _____.

8. _____ is loss of memory.

9. An incision into the skull is called _____.

10. _____ is throat spasms caused by the sight of water or attempting to drink water.

Use the words in the list to complete the following statements:

status epilepticus   shingles

quadriplegia   encephalitis

pia mater   nuchal rigidity

paraplegia   Parkinson's disease

dura mater, arachnoid, pia mater   central

11. Constant jerky uncontrollable movement is called _____.

12. _____ is an abnormal sensation, burning, tingling, or numbness.

13. Paralysis of all four extremities is called _____.

14. Inflammation of the brain is called _____.

15. _____ _____ is the inner layer of the meninges.

16. _____ _____ is a condition where the neck resists bending forward or sideways.

17. Paralysis below the waist is called _____.

18. Pill-rolling of the fingers is a classic symptom of _____ _____.

19. The brain and the spinal cord make up the _____ nervous system.

20. The three layers of the meninges are called the _____, _____, and _____.

Use the words in the list to complete the following statements:

amyotrophic lateral sclerosis   Bell's palsy

electroencephalogram   epilepsy

headaches   multiple sclerosis

shingles   sleep apnea

spinal fluid   status epilepticus

21. The circulating fluid in the brain and spinal cord is called _____ _____.

22. A(n) _____ is a procedure to evaluate electrical brain activity.

23. _____ is a disease caused by the virus herpes zoster.

24. Tension, cluster, and migraine are types of _____.

25. A chronic disease of the brain characterized by intermittent episodes of abnormal electrical activity is called _____.

26. _____ _____ is a state of continued convulsive seizure with no recovery of consciousness.

27. A disease causing unilateral paralysis of the face is called _____.

28. A sleep disorder characterized by periods of apnea or breathlessness is called _____ _____.

29. Demyelination of the nerves of the central nervous system is called _____ _____.

30. A destructive disease of the motor neurons is called _____ _____ _____.

Short Answer

Provide answers to the following:

1. Describe components of the nervous system.

   _____

   _____

   _____

2. What are the common signs and symptoms of nervous system disorders?

   _____

   _____

   _____

3. List the cranial nerves and their function(s).

   a. _____

   b. _____

   c. _____

   d. _____

   e. _____

   f. _____

   g. _____

   h. _____

   i. _____

   j. _____

   k. _____

   l. _____

4. Describe the spinal nerves.

_____

_____

_____

True / False

_____ 1. Immunosuppressed individuals must follow precautions with polio vaccines.

_____ 2. Dr. Jonas Salk developed an oral vaccine against all three forms of virus called a trivalent vaccine (TOPV—Trivalent Oral Polio Vaccine).

_____ 3. There are three distinct polioviruses designated as types 1, 2, and 3.

_____ 4. A recently researched cost-saving treatment for headaches is acupuncture.

_____ 5. Acupuncture treatment for headaches only works well on children with chronic headaches.

_____ 6. The traditional Chinese method of using acupuncture for migraine headaches was not found to be an effective treatment.

_____ 7. A seizure is a sign of a malfunction of some part of the brain's electrical system.

_____ 8. Most seizures in individuals diagnosed with epilepsy are not emergencies.

CASE STUDY

Joseph is an 80-year-old grandfather of six children. The ages of his grandchildren range from 11 to 35. At a recent family reunion, several of them stated concern about their grandfather's decreasing functioning. They were told this is a typical occurrence in aging.

What are the normal effects of aging on the nervous system?

_____

_____

_____

CHAPTER 16

Eye and Ear Diseases and Disorders

Define Terms

Define the following terms:

1. cerumen _____

   _____

2. diplopia _____

   _____

3. ophthalmoscope _____

   _____

4. otoscope _____

   _____

5. otalgia _____

   _____

6. tonometry _____

   _____

7. stapedectomy _____

   _____

8. vertigo _____

   _____

9. myringotomy _____

   _____

10. pruritis _____

    _____

Matching

Match the following terms with the correct definition:

1. amblyopia
2. enucleation
3. mastoidectomy
4. photophobia
5. pruritis

A. itching
B. fear of light
C. removal of the eyeball
D. caused by a pathogen or a disease
E. removal of the mastoid bone
F. decrease in vision due to lack of stimuli

Match the following terms with the correct definition:

6. suppurative
7. tinnitus
8. topical
9. tympanoplasty
10. purulent

A. placed on the skin
B. formation of pus
C. surgical repair of the eardrum
D. ringing in the ears
E. referring to the entire body
F. full of dead neutrophils and bacteria

Identify Diagnostic Tests

Explain the following tests:

1. ophthalmoscopy _____
2. visual acuity measurement _____
3. tonometry _____
4. slit-lamp examination _____
5. angiography _____
6. otoscopic examination _____
7. audiometry _____

Condition Table

Complete the following table:

Condition and Definition	Signs and Symptoms	Diagnostic Tests	Treatment Plan
Retinal Detachment			
Otosclerosis			
Diabetic Retinopathy			
Mastoiditis			
Otitis Media			

Ménière's Disease			
Cataracts			
Strabismus			
Macular Degeneration			

Completion

Use the words in the list below to complete the following:

anterior chamber   pinna
choroid layer   pupil
cornea   retina
iris   sclera
lens   tympanic membrane

1. _____ is also known as the outer ear.
2. The clear fibers enclosed in a membrane that refract and focus light to the retina are called the _____.
3. _____ is also known as the eardrum.
4. The clear tissue that covers the pupil and iris is called the _____.
5. _____ is the inside layer of the posterior part of the eye that receives light rays.
6. The layer between the sclera and the retina containing blood vessels is called the _____ _____.
7. _____ is the round disk of muscles that gives the eye its color.
8. The white area covering the outside of the eye except over the pupil and iris is called the _____.
9. _____ is the round opening in the iris that changes its size as the iris reacts to light and dark.
10. The space between the cornea and the iris is called the _____ _____.

Short Answer

Please provide answers to the following:

1. List the anatomical components of the eyes.

_____
_____
_____

2. List the anatomical components of the ear.

_____
_____
_____

3. Which cranial nerves innervate the eye?

_____

_____

_____

5. How does the ear help the body maintain equilibrium?

_____

_____

_____

6. What are some common signs and symptoms of eye disorders?

_____

_____

_____

7. What are some common signs and symptoms of ear disorders?

_____

_____

_____

True / False

_____   1. Dry eye syndrome can be helped by eating a healthy diet.

_____   2. Antioxidants are agents that can be naturally found in vegetables, fruits, and plants.

_____   3. When irrigating the ear, you should use a bulb syringe filled with hot water.

_____   4. Impacted cerumen in the ear should be softened and removed gently.

_____   5. There have been some promising results from using vascular endothelial growth factor (VEGF) treatment of age-related macular degeneration (AMD).

_____   6. Vascular endothelial growth factor belongs to the family of drugs called angiogenesis inhibitors.

_____   7. Angiogenesis inhibitors are agents that help blood vessel growth.

_____   8. Vitamins C and E are the antioxidant vitamins.

CASE STUDY

Lilly is a 67-year-old retired teacher. She has noticed blurring and decreasing vision over the past few months. She visited her ophthalmologist, who diagnosed her with cataracts. She is concerned about the condition of her eyes and eventual treatment of the cataracts.

What is the expected treatment for Lilly's condition?

_____

_____

CHAPTER 17

Reproductive System Diseases and Disorders

Defining Terms

Define the following terms:

1. amenorrhea _____

_____

2. leukorrhea _____

_____

3. chancre _____

_____

4. epididymitis _____

_____

5. septicemia _____

_____

6. vaginitis _____

_____

7. prophylactic _____

_____

8. ectopic _____

_____

9. primigravid _____

_____

10. antiemetic _____

_____

Matching

Match the following terms with the correct definition:

1. prepuce
2. dysmenorrhea
3. menorrhagia
4. metrorrhagia
5. dyspareunia

A. state of being inactive
B. painful menses
C. excessive menses
D. excessive bleeding between menstrual periods
E. painful sexual intercourse
F. foreskin

Match the following terms with the correct definition:

6. leiomyomas
7. multiparity
8. proteinuria
9. uterine prolapse
10. mammoplasty

A. surgical reconstruction of the breasts
B. uterus drops or protrudes downward
C. protein or albumin in the urine
D. multiple births
E. benign tumors of the uterus
F. white vaginal discharge

Define Abbreviations

Define the following abbreviations:

1. VDRL _____

_____

2. D&C _____

_____

3. PID _____

_____

4. PMS _____

_____

5. BPH _____

_____

6. STD _____

_____

7. AIDS _____

_____

8. TURP _____

_____

Identify Diagnostic Tests

Define the following diagnostic tests:

1. laparoscopy _____

_____

2. hysterosalpingogram _____

_____

3. bimanual examination _____

_____

4. cytological _____

_____

5. mammogram _____

_____

6. digital rectal examination _____

_____

7. Pap smear _____

_____

8. culture and sensitivity _____

_____

9. prostatic specific antigen _____

_____

Condition Table

Complete the following table:

Disease Condition and Definition	Signs and Symptoms	Diagnostic Tests	Treatment Plan
Transurethral Resection of the Prostate			
Ectopic Pregnancy			
Hyperemesis Gravidarum			
Abruptio Placentae			
Placenta Previa			
Toxic Shock Syndrome			
Menopause			

(Continued)

Disease Condition and Definition	Signs and Symptoms	Diagnostic Tests	Treatment Plan
Mastectomy			
Premenstrual Syndrome			
Endometriosis			

Completion

Use the words in the list to complete the following statements:

amenorrhea	endometriosis
dyspareunia	metrorrhagia
dysmenorrhea	menorrhagia
hysterosalpingogram	laparoscopy
cytology	prepuce
spontaneous abortion	hyperemesis

1. _____ means without menses.

2. Abnormal growth of the lining of the uterus outside the uterus is called _____.

3. _____ is painful sexual intercourse.

4. Abnormal bleeding between menstrual periods is called _____.

5. Bad, painful, or difficult menses is known as _____.

6. _____ is excessive or prolonged menstrual bleeding.

7. An X-ray of the uterus and the fallopian tubes is called a(n) _____.

8. A procedure done to look inside the abdominal cavity is called a(n) _____.

9. The study of cells is called _____.

10. The medical term for the foreskin is _____.

11. _____ _____ is commonly known as a miscarriage.

12. _____ is excessive vomiting.

Use the words in the list to complete the following statements:

chancre	digital rectal examination
syphilis	menopause
mastectomy	cervicitis
clap	cryptorchidism
ectopic pregnancy	epididymitis
hysterosalpingogram	orchidectomy
pre-eclampsia	primigravida

13. Another name for toxemia is _____.

14. The medical term for first pregnancy is _____.

15. A pregnancy that occurs when the fertilized ovum attaches outside the uterus is called _____.

16. Surgical excision of the testes is called a(n) _____ _____

17. _____ is undescended testicles.

18. Inflammation of the storage tank for sperm is called _____.

19. The slang word for gonorrhea is _____.

20. A painless, highly contagious lesion is called _____.

21. In order to feel the prostate, the physician must perform a _____ _____ _____.

22. A VDRL and an RPR are blood tests performed to test for _____.

23. The natural halting of menstruation is called _____.

24. The surgical excision of the breast is called _____.

25. Inflammation of the cervix is called _____.

Short Answer

Provide answers to the following:

1. List the components of the reproductive system.

   Female:

   _____

   _____

   Male:

   _____

   _____

2. What are the common signs and symptoms of reproductive system disorders?

   Female:

   _____

   _____

   Male:

   _____

   _____

3. Explain the following procedures:

   lumpectomy _____

   _____

   mastectomy _____

   _____

   mammoplasty _____

   _____

panhysterectomy _____

_____

orchiectomy _____

_____

transurethral resection of the prostate _____

_____

A&P repair _____

_____

cystoscopy _____

_____

hysterectomy _____

_____

D&C _____

_____

True / False

_____ 1. Tamoxifen is a drug that is frequently used for the treatment of breast cancer.

_____ 2. Recently, researchers have been looking at the use of taurine (an organic acid found mostly in bile but also in other tissues in the body) to overcome some of the serious side effects of tamoxifen.

_____ 3. It is quite common to find cases of lead poisoning in persons who have taken herbal preparations for infertility.

_____ 4. The public should be aware that unbranded herbal products should be avoided or taken with extreme caution.

⟳ CASE STUDY

Susie and **Jim** have been married for 8 years and have been unable to conceive a child. They have talked about this on a couple occasions with their family physician but have not really done anything about it to this point in time. They would like to know more about infertility and what treatments are available.

1. What are some of the causes of infertility?

_____

_____

2. What treatment options are available that Susie and Jim might investigate?

_____

_____

CHAPTER 18

Integumentary System Diseases and Disorders

Defining Terms

Define the following terms:

1. abrasion _____

_____

2. comedones _____

_____

3. erythema _____

_____

4. lesion _____

_____

5. pruritus _____

_____

6. sebum _____

_____

7. vesicles _____

_____

8. pustules _____

_____

9. keratin _____

_____

10. ulcer _____

_____

Matching

Match the disease with the correct definition:

____	1. seborrheic dermatitis of an infant	A. "seven-year itch"
____	2. eczema	B. shingles
____	3. scleroderma	C. cellulitis of the face caused by strep
____	4. erysipelas	D. chickenpox
____	5. pediculosis	E. atopic dermatitis
____	6. scabies	F. inflammation and infection of the hair follicle
____	7. tinea pedis	G. hardening of the skin
____	8. folliculitis	H. athlete's foot
____	9. herpes varicella	I. lice
____	10. herpes zoster	J. "cradle cap"

Identify Diagnostic Tests

Define the following diagnostic tests:

1. culture and sensitivity _____

_____

2. skin scrapings _____

_____

3. incision and drainage (I&D) _____

_____

4. curettage _____

_____

5. biopsy _____

_____

Condition Table

Complete the following table:

Condition and Definition	Signs and Symptoms	Diagnostic Tests	Treatment Plan
Herpes			
Impetigo			
Abscess, Furuncle, Carbuncle			
Lyme Disease			

Tinea Pedis			
Candidiasis			
Pediculosis			
Acne			
Seborrheic Dermatitis			
Eczema			
Psoriasis			
Malignant Melanoma			
Burns: First-, Second-, and Third-Degree			
Decubitus Ulcer			
Corns and Calluses			
Ringworm			

Completion

Using the words in the list, complete the following statements:

abrasion	pilonidal cyst
comedone	pruritus
erythema	pustule
lesion	sebum
paronychia	ulcer
papule	wheal

1. _____ is produced by the sebaceous glands.

2. _____ is the medical term for redness.

3. Severe itching is also known as _____.

4. A broad term meaning abnormality of tissue or any discontinuity is called a(n) _____.

5. A(n) _____ is a small circumscribed elevation of the skin containing pus.

6. A small solid raised lesion less than 0.5 cm in diameter is called a(n) _____.

7. A(n) _____ is an open sore or erosion of the skin or mucous membrane.

8. A smooth, slightly elevated, swollen area that is redder or paler than the surrounding skin is usually accompanied by itching is known as a(n) _____.

9. A(n) _____ is a plugged skin pore.

10. A type of sebaceous cyst is called a _____.

11. Bacterial infection of the nails is called a(n) _____.

12. A common mechanical injury caused by scraping away the skin surface is called a(n) _____.

Using the words in the list, complete the statements below:

avulsion	ephilis
blunt trauma	nevus
laceration	hirsutism
vesicles	alopecia
pressure ulcer	hemangioma
hematoma	cradle cap

13. A(n) _____ occurs when a portion of skin or an appendage is pulled or torn away.

14. A cut in the skin caused by a sharp object such as a knife, razor, or glass is known medically as a(n) _____.

15. When an individual is struck by an item such as a hammer or club or is thrown into an object like a steering wheel or wall, the individual may sustain a _____ _____ injury.

16. _____ are fluid-filled circumscribed elevations.

17. A decubitus ulcer is also called a(n) _____.

18. A large bruise is called a(n) _____.

19. _____ is a freckle.

20. A(n) _____ is the same as a mole.

21. _____ is excessive hair growth.

22. Complete or partial hair loss is called _____.

23. A benign tumor of the blood vessels is called a(n) _____.

24. Infant seborrheic dermatitis is called _____.

Using the words in the list, complete the statements below:

chickenpox	verruca
epidermis	urticaria
erysipelas	shingles
folliculitis	lice
frostbite	keloid
herpes simplex II	jock itch

25. Hives are also called _____.

26. Tinea cruris is commonly known as _____.

27. A strep cellulitis of the face is called _____.

28. Pediculosis is also called _____.

29. Inflammation and infection of a hair follicle is _____.

30. Herpes zoster is also known as _____.

31. Herpes varicella is commonly called _____.

32. The _____ is the outer layer of skin.

33. _____ is also known as warts.

34. Genital herpes is also known as _____.

35. A(n) _____ is a raised, firm, irregular-shaped mass of scar tissue that develops following trauma or surgical incision.

36. Freezing of tissue usually on the face, fingers, toes, and ears is called _____.

Short Answer

Please provide answers to the following:

1. Describe the skin.

2. List the common signs and symptoms of skin problems.

3. What are the various types of herpes?

    a. _____

    b. _____

    c. _____

    d. _____

True / False

_____ 1. Lysine is a beneficial treatment for herpes genitalis.

_____ 2. Several research studies have shown traditional Chinese medicine to be beneficial for psoriasis and atopic dermatitis.

_____ 3. Using sunscreen with an SPF of 30 or higher on all exposed skin is recommended to prevent sunburn.

_____ 4. Using tanning beds is a good method for tanning the skin without harm.

CASE STUDY

1. **John** is 32 years old and has been diagnosed with AIDS. He has also been diagnosed with Kaposi's sarcoma.

   A. Why is John more likely to get Kaposi's sarcoma than anyone else?

   _____

   _____

   B. What symptoms would you expect John to present with?

   _____

   _____

   C. What is the treatment for Kaposi's sarcoma?

   _____

   _____

2. **Debra Smith** has noticed a dark-colored area on her left arm. She first noticed this area 3–4 weeks ago. The area seems to be getting darker and the shape of the area has changed recently. The physician has diagnosed Debra with malignant melanoma.

   A. Where does this tumor usually metastasize?

   _____

   B. What risk factors might Debra have for developing melanoma?

   _____

   _____

   _____

   C. How is melanoma diagnosed?

   _____

   _____

   D. What is the prognosis for melanoma?

   _____

   _____

   _____

Genetic/ Developmental, Childhood, and Mental Health Diseases and Disorders

Genetic and Developmental Diseases and Disorders

Defining Terms

Define the following terms:

1. anomaly _____

_____

2. atresia _____

_____

3. dystrophy _____

_____

4. autosomes _____

_____

5. congenital _____

_____

6. dominant _____

_____

7. exocrine _____

_____

8. gene _____

_____

9. genotype _____

_____

10. somatic _____

_____

Matching

Match the following terms with the correct definition:

1. buccal smear
2. epicanthus
3. heterozygous
4. karyotyping
5. microcephaly

A. having different paired genes

B. a test for evaluating chromosomes utilizing cells from the mouth

C. a unit on the chromosome

D. a method of identifying chromosomes

E. a fold of skin across the medial aspect of the eye

F. an abnormally small head

Match the following terms with the correct definition:

6. mitosis
7. recessive
8. stricture
9. viscous
10. pyloromyotomy

A. reproduction of cells that yields identical daughter cells

B. thick

C. weak, lacks control

D. surgery on a sphincter muscle of the stomach

E. narrowing

F. part of the chromosome carrying DNA

Define Abbreviations

Define the following abbreviations:

1. FAS _____

_____

2. PKU _____

_____

3. CP _____

_____

4. CHD _____

_____

5. MD _____

_____

Identify Diagnostic Tests

Identify the following diagnostic tests:

1. amniotic fluid analysis _____

_____

2. ultrasonography _____

_____

3. muscle biopsy _____

_____

4. electromyography _____

_____

5. blood test for phenylketonuria _____

_____

Condition Table

Complete the following table:

Condition and Definition	Signs and Symptoms	Diagnostic Tests	Treatment Plan
Tay-Sachs Disease			
Fetal Alcohol Syndrome			
Hirschsprung's Disease			
Down Syndrome			
Phenylketonuria			
Failure to Thrive			
Imperforate Anus			
Cleft Palate			
Tetralogy of Fallot			
Meckel's Diverticulum			

Completion

Use the following words to complete the statements below:

anomaly	auscultation
blue babies	dominant
congenital	germ cells
murmur	phenotype
microencephaly	imperforate anus
karyotyping	Meckel's diverticulum

1. Babies born with tetralogy of Fallot are called _____ _____.

2. An abnormality is known as a(n) _____.

3. A condition a person is born with is known as _____.

4. An abnormal heart sound is called a(n) _____.

5. _____ is a small brain.

6. The process of visualizing chromosomes is called _____.

7. _____ is listening to the chest with a stethoscope.

8. A gene in control is a _____ gene.

9. _____ are also called sex cells.

10. The expression of a trait such as brown hair or blue eyes is called a(n) _____.

11. Failure of the anus to connect to the rectum is called _____.

12. Outpouching of the diverticulum of the ileum is known as _____ _____.

Use the following words to complete the statements below:

coarctation of the aorta	harelip
phenylketonuria	chordee
failure to thrive	hydrocephalus
talipes equinovarus	atrial septal defect
Tay-Sachs	FAS
anencephaly	atresia
gene	

13. _____ _____ is the narrowing of the descending thoracic aorta.

14. A cleft lip is also called a(n) _____.

15. Faulty protein metabolism causes a disease called _____.

16. Abnormal downward curvature of the penis is known as _____.

17. _____ _____ is lack of physical growth and development in an infant or child.

18. _____ is water on the brain.

19. Clubfoot is known medically as _____.

20. An opening between the right and left atria is called _____ _____ _____.

21. _____ is an error in lipid metabolism and results in an accumulation of toxins in the brain.

22. The abbreviation for fetal alcohol syndrome is _____.

23. Severe congenital malformation resulting in the absence of the brain or cranial vault is called _____.

24. Congenital absence or closure of a normal opening or lumen in the body is known as _____.

25. A(n) _____ is an ultramicroscopic unit of DNA.

Short Answer

Please provide answers to the following:

1. Describe chromosomes.

_____

_____

_____

_____

2. Describe how genetic disorders are passed to offspring from parents.

 a. _____

 b. _____

 c. _____

 d. _____

3. What are the causes of congenital anomalies?

 a. _____

 b. _____

 c. _____

 d. _____

True / False

____ 1. A variety of herbal preparations and supplements, such as creatine, glutamine, and green tea extract, have been used to treat muscular dystrophy and related disorders.

____ 2. Problems with hypertonicity in cerebral palsy may be lessened using botulinum toxin A.

____ 3. Botulinum toxin A is the same as botox, which is used in dermatology.

____ 4. Duchenne's muscular dystrophy is now routinely treated successfully with an "antisense" compound.

____ 5. In Duchenne's muscular dystrophy, the individual overproduces the essential muscle protein called dystrophin.

CASE STUDY

Mr. and **Mrs. Pearson** have three children who are grown. Two years ago they were surprised when they found out Mrs. Pearson was pregnant again. After birth, their daughter Casey was diagnosed with Down syndrome. She is a loving child but does have some limitations.

What are some of the typical signs of Down syndrome?

_____

_____

_____

_____

_____

_____

_____

Childhood Diseases and Disorders

Define Terms

Define the following terms:

1. incubation period _____

    _____

2. malaise _____

    _____

3. Koplik's spots _____

    _____

4. rhinitis _____

    _____

5. catarrhal _____

    _____

6. paroxysmal _____

    _____

7. pyoderma _____

    _____

8. inspiratory stridor _____

    _____

9. supine _____

    _____

10. prone _____

    _____

11. colic _____

    _____

12. intrathecal _____

    _____

13. exudates _____

_____

14. flatulence _____

_____

15. nits _____

_____

Matching

Match the following terms with the correct definition:

_____ 1. dormant

_____ 2. encephalopathy

_____ 3. euphoric

_____ 4. orchitis

_____ 5. adenoidectomy

A. a sense of well-being

B. surgical removal of the adnoids

C. state of being inactive

D. inflammation of the testis

E. disease of the brain

F. listening to the heart with a stethoscope

Match the following terms with the correct definition:

_____ 6. tonsillectomy

_____ 7. vesicles

_____ 8. patent

_____ 9. hallucinogenic

_____ 10. parotid glands

A. blister-like eruptions on the skin

B. producing psychedelic alterations in function

C. salivary glands

D. surgery to remove tissue in the nasopharynx

E. open

F. a state of ill feeling

Define Abbreviations

Define the following abbreviations:

1. AIDS _____

_____

2. HIV _____

_____

3. SIDS _____

_____

4. TB _____

_____

5. MMR _____

_____

6. DTP –hib _____

_____

Identify Diagnostic Tests

Identify the following diagnostic tests:

1. chest X-ray _____

_____

2. sputum culture _____

_____

3. skin tests _____

_____

4. throat culture _____

_____

5. stool examination _____

_____

6. pulmonary function tests _____

_____

7. bone scan _____

_____

8. bone marrow biopsy _____

_____

9. complete blood count _____

_____

10. audiometry _____

_____

Condition Table

Complete the following table:

Condition and Definition	Signs and Symptoms	Diagnostic Tests	Treatment Plan
Tonsillitis			
Sudden Infant Death Syndrome			
Measles			
Mumps			
Rubella			
Pertussis			

(Continued)

Condition and Definition	Signs and Symptoms	Diagnostic Tests	Treatment Plan
Diphtheria			
AIDS			
Croup			
Tuberculosis			

Completion

Use the words in the list to complete the following statements:

rubeola	mumps
whooping cough	orchitis
influenza	rubella
flatulence	catarrhal
vesicles	malaise

1. Another name for measles is _____.

2. Pertussis is also called _____.

3. An infection of the parotid glands is known as _____.

4. An inflammation of the testes is called _____.

5. _____ is more commonly called the flu.

6. _____ are unique to measles and are often the definitive symptom that make the diagnosis.

7. _____ is excessive gas.

8. _____ are blister-like eruptions on the skin.

9. Inflammation of the nasal mucous membranes is called _____.

10. _____ is a feeling of general discomfort.

Use the words in the list to complete the following statements:

dormant	paroxysmal
incubation period	prone
inspiratory stridor	strabismus
laryngotracheobronchitis	supine
nits	tularemia

11. The _____ _____ is the time between exposure to the disease and the presence of the symptoms that lasts several days.

12. _____ _____ is a high-pitched sound during inspiration due to a blocked airway.

13. _____ is a spasm or convulsion.

14. _____ is the state of being inactive.

15. _____ are lice eggs.

16. _____ is lying face down.

17. _____ is lying face up.

18. Rabbit fever is also known as _____.

19. _____ is also known as croup.

20. A crossed or lazy eye is called _____.

Short Answer

Please provide answers to the following:

1. What is the recommended schedule for immunizations for children?

_____

_____

_____

_____

_____

_____

2. Describe some important points about respiratory diseases in children.

_____

_____

_____

_____

3. Describe some important points about fungal diseases in children.

_____

_____

_____

_____

4. Describe some important points about digestive diseases in children.

_____

_____

_____

_____

5. Describe some important points about viral diseases in children.

_____

_____

_____

_____

True / False

_____ 1. There have been several clinical trials studying complementary and alternative medicine (CAM) therapy for upper respiratory tract infections in children.

_____ 2. Vitamin C and homeopathic medicines are very effective for treating respiratory problems in children.

_____ 3. It is okay to tell children that medicine is candy.

_____ 4. Mouthwash is not harmful to children.

_____ 5. Some plants commonly found in the home can be toxic to children.

_____ 6. Child-resistant packaging does not mean childproof packaging.

_____ 7. The meningococcal vaccine is only recommended for adults.

_____ 8. The varicella vaccine is given to prevent chickenpox.

CASE STUDY

Nancy is the mother of **Jamie,** a toddler who seems to be very curious. Nancy is concerned about the safety of her home with a toddler who is very active and can wander throughout the one-level home rather easily. Besides putting all medicines, cosmetics, and plants out of Jamie's reach, what other tips should Nancy know about preventing poisonings in children?

_____

_____

_____

_____

_____

_____

_____

CHAPTER 21

Mental Health Diseases and Disorders

Define Terms

Define the following terms:

1. addiction _____

   _____

2. affect _____

   _____

3. bulimia _____

   _____

4. delirium tremens _____

   _____

5. circadian rhythms _____

   _____

6. delusions _____

   _____

7. dependency _____

   _____

8. intoxicated _____

   _____

9. mania _____

   _____

10. tolerance _____

    _____

Matching

Match the following terms with the correct definition:

_____ 1. obsession

_____ 2. organic

_____ 3. stuttering

_____ 4. enuresis

_____ 5. tics

A. a speech problem

B. related to an organ or physical component

C. sudden, rapid muscle movement or vocalization

D. hyperactivity disorder

E. commonly called *bedwetting*

F. repetition of a thought or emotion

Match the following terms with the correct definition:

_____ 6. narcotics

_____ 7. phychosis

_____ 8. schizophrenia

_____ 9. grandiose

_____ 10. malingering

A. depressants used as analgesics or painkillers

B. disintergration of one's personality and loss of contact with reality

C. fictitious display of symptoms in order to gain a reward

D. "split mind," a serious mental condition

E. inflated sense of self-worth

F. suspicious actions and feelings

Define Abbreviations

Define the following abbreviations:

1. OCD _____

_____

2. PTSD _____

_____

3. SAD _____

_____

4. ADHD _____

_____

5. AA _____

_____

6. DTs _____

_____

Condition Table

Complete the following table:

Condition and Definition	Signs and Symptoms	Diagnostic Tests	Treatment Plan
Anorexia			
Bulimia			

Autism			
Schizophrenia			
Intellectual Disability			
Attention-Deficit Hyperactivity Disorder			
Alcoholism			
Depression			
Seasonal Affective Disorder			
Personality Disorders			
Munchausen Syndrome			
Bipolar Disease			

Completion

Use the words in the list to complete the following statements:

delusion	addiction
stuttering	intoxication
affective disorders	mania
organic	tolerance
withdrawal	tics
bedwetting	psychoses
jealousy	

1. A false belief that is firmly adhered to although it is not shared by others is a _____.

2. _____ is the physical or psychological dependence on a substance.

3. Stammering is also known as _____.

4. _____ occurs when blood alcohol levels reach 0.10 percent or more.

5. Disorders that involve emotions are called _____ _____.

6. Extreme elation or agitation is known as _____.

7. Mental disorders with some type of known physical cause are called _____.

8. _____ is the ability to endure large amounts of a substance without an adverse effect.

9. Unpleasant physical and psychological effects resulting from stopping the use of a substance after the individual is addicted are called _____.

10. _____ are sudden, rapid muscle movements or vocalization.

11. _____ is medically known as *enuresis*.

12. _____ are characterized by a disintegration of one's personality and loss of contact with reality.

13. _____ is the belief that one's sexual partner is unfaithful.

Use the words in the list to complete the following statements:

exhibitionism	voyeurism
grief	transvestic
histrionic	schizophrenia
multiple	schizoid
narcolepsy	panic disorder
paranoid	winter
pedophilia	

14. "Split mind" or split personality is also known as _____.

15. Seasonal affective disorder is also known as _____ depression.

16. A _____ _____ is also called a panic attack.

17. Individuals exhibiting two or more distinct personalities are said to have _____ personalities.

18. A _____ personality exhibits traits of jealousy, suspicion, envy, and hypersensitivity.

19. Loners have _____ personalities.

20. Individuals with a _____ personality may be overly dramatic with expressions of their emotions.

21. _____ occurs when males expose their genitals to an unsuspecting female.

22. The person who is aroused by cross-dressing is said to have _____ fetishism.

23. The person who is sexually aroused by children is called _____.

24. _____ involves arousal by secretly watching others undress or engage in sexual activity; individuals with this condition are often called "Peeping Toms."

25. Daily uncontrollable attack of sleep is called _____.

26. _____ is the natural process of coping with loss.

Short Answer

Please provide answers to the following:

1. What are some common signs and symptoms of mental health disorders?

_____

_____

_____

2. What are some categories of common mental health disorders?

_____

_____

_____

_____

3. What are some genetic and acquired causes of intellectual disability?

_____

_____

_____

_____

True / False

_____ 1. An early diagnosis of Alzheimer's disease makes a significant difference in the prognosis.

_____ 2. In recent studies, researchers are looking at using cerebrospinal fluid biomarkers to find Alzheimer's disease in individuals.

_____ 3. Lemon balm is a perennial herb found in the mint family.

_____ 4. Lemon balm has been effective in the treatment of severe Alzheimer's disease.

CASE STUDY

Jeffrey is a 43-year-old male who was recently laid off from his job in the auto industry. His wife is concerned that he will become clinically depressed if he cannot get back to work soon.

What are some of the characteristics of depression that Jeffrey's wife might observe?

_____

_____

_____

_____